TABLE OF CONTENTS

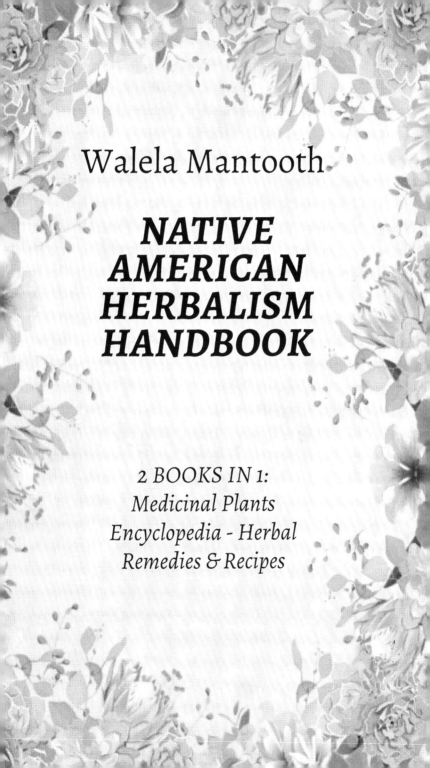

Walela Mantooth

NATIVE AMERICAN HERBALISM HANDBOOK

2 BOOKS IN 1:
*Medicinal Plants
Encyclopedia - Herbal
Remedies & Recipes*

This book is dedicated to my grandfather who unfortunately is no longer with us

He taught me everything I know about native American herbal medicine practices that I still use today

I decided to honor my grandfather by writing this book with the intention of passing on to as many people as possible this knowledge about plants and herbs which have been used for centuries by our Native Americans

Thanks grandpa you are the real author of this book!

Introduction

For thousands of years, man has made use of alternative medicine to cure illnesses, fight viruses, and find solutions to stubborn diseases. These methods have been carefully developed, researched, and preserved so they can be useful for generations to come. Then came modern civilization and its complexity that brought us further and further from nature. Everything changed, and much of the old wisdom was forgotten.

Native American medicine used to be a very important part of human existence in Northern America. It was vital for the people as it ensured their health and ability to fight off infections. Then came modern medicine, and people came to disdain these natural remedies that existed and were effective long ago. Instead of free and natural medicines provided by the earth, the desire to make huge profits from people's illness has now become the major impetus behind our medical system.

In recent years, people are beginning to investigate if humans can benefit from the lifestyle of people who existed hundreds and even thousands of years ago. Based on research, these peoples had fewer medical problems compared to what we have today and were able to have good health with very little resources.

Did these Native American people know what we do not know now? What is it that we can learn from them? Do they have the answers to some of the most dangerous health problems that we have today, including cancer, Ebola, and HIV/AIDS?

Native Americans understood the interconnected nature of all life and the truth that a human's well-being depended on the mind, body, and spirit being in harmony. An imbalance in any one of the three and illness results. These ancient people, through their close connection to the natural world, discovered that certain plants could heal certain imbalances in the human body.

Through their collective learning, Native Americans cataloged over 500 different plants and their medicinal uses. What makes this knowledge even more amazing is that this was all done through oral tradition as their knowledge was not written down until modern times.

Despite all of the knowledge and technology at our disposal, modern medicine has very serious limitations. If it didn't, we would not be spending billions every year treating illnesses and diseases that are far more prevalent now than in the past.

Perhaps what modern medicine is missing is a more holistic, nature-based way of approaching health and healing.

In this book, you will learn how to look for and find the perfect Native American medicines. You will receive guidance on how to work with skilled professionals and the benefits you will derive from using a medicine that is in harmony with nature. You will also learn how using native medicine can help reduce the cost of your medical expenses.

The world of Native American herbal medicine is vast and deeply enriching for those who take the time to explore its treasures.

You may enjoy your exploration and, with the help of this book, gain the knowledge needed to heal yourself.

,

Chapter 1

Introduction to Native American Culture

Native Americans have healing traditions that can be traced back for literally thousands of years, and there were many tribes who had their own ways to mix the roots, herbs, and other plant parts that were meant to heal their people. Though, that doesn't mean only herbs were used in the healing process Native Americans found.

No healing practice was the same when you go tribe from tribe, but you will see that they have many similarities in their ceremonies, knowledge, and rituals. There was no standard of healing, but health was an expression of the spirit to Native American people. They believed that you had to heal the spirit, the mind, and the body, or someone would not make it through. It was important to them to stick to their natural environment to keep away illness and harm that may come their way. Of course, they also knew that they had to heal their physical ailments as well if they really wanted to get better.

The main part of these healing practices was the herbal remedies that came with them, and it went beyond the aches and pains of the body. Of course, while they concentrated on the physical ailment, they also told the patient it was important to concentrate on their spirituality and the harmony within themselves as well, giving many Native Americans the will to survive through various afflictions.

The surrounding environment would produce the herbs that they used, which meant that there was a diverse number of cures that varied from region to region. They were even traded over long distances, as herbs were considered to be valuable and even sacred. The practices were passed down orally, and it went from generation to generation without writing it down. This is why many of the healing remedies today are still a mystery, but some healers would end up writing down their own formulas for healing as well.

Today, many of the herbs that were used are known, and many of the purposes they had and still have been seen. However, that doesn't mean that everything is crystal clear as it would have been years ago when it was being passed down from one person to the next.

KNOWING IF NATIVE AMERICAN MEDICINE CAN HELP

This is something that is usually needing to be discussed with a medical professional. Of course, you will find that some herbs are able to be used in conjunction with other medications, and they will help you to feel a little better. Though, it isn't just the herbs that will help you. There are still many Native American healing remedies that will help you to understand your body, spirituality, and your path to healing. Though, it is always important that you consult a medical professional before you start using any Native American medicine or healing practice.

Self-diagnosing doesn't help anyone, and you need to make sure that herbs are safe to use with the medicine, over-the-counter, or prescription, that you may be taking. Herbs can even interact with one another, so it is important that a medical professional helps you decide if Native American healing is an alternative medicine source that can help you.

Before you can learn anything about how to use medicinal herbs, it is crucial that you first understand herbal medicine and its history.

So, before anything, let us define what a medicinal herb is. A medicinal herb is a plant that has characteristics that are identical to that of a modern pharmaceutical drug. Essentially, what this means is that they are plants that bear healing power, in the same way that modern medicines do.

You can find plants that can treat headaches, colds, allergies, and other medical problems just as you would find appropriate drugs for the same. In a way, they act as healthy alternatives.

On the other hand, pharmaceutical drugs are different because they are manufactured in laboratories. They serve the same purpose but are produced differently, often through a combination of plant extracts and other chemicals.

It is safe to state that herbal medicine is not a relatively new thing to mankind. Herbal medicine has been around for ages. Evidence from archaeology suggests the use of herbal medicine approximately 60,000 years ago. It was a common belief that plants had both magical and healing powers. Then at around 500 B.C, people started perceiving sickness as a natural condition in humans, which led to the abandonment of superstitious beliefs.

In the 14th century, people started trading medicinal herbs in the world trade that was popular at the time. This exchange happened primarily between the Europeans, Indians, Chinese, and Arabs. Herbs like cinnamon, ginger, and cardamom were introduced to Europe around this time.

In the period between the twelfth and

eighteenth century, various illnesses spread across Europe and the drugs at the time proved ineffective at combating them. Later on, the Spanish and Portuguese landed in Central America and began developing an herbal medicine that would counter the illnesses in Europe.

These medicines were effective and were used widely to treat malaria, smallpox, syphilis, and other rampant illnesses. It was around this time that herbal medicine gained massive popularity. To this day, herbal medicine is still popular in some parts of this world, especially areas where modern medicine may not be readily available such as Africa.

Chapter 2

Herbal Remedies for Your Child

Here is a list of essential herbs and the age groups most appropriate for them. Starting with newborns, you can add the essential oils to the list of the other age groups, but you cannot add them in regression.

0-2 MONTH

NEWBORN DILL [ANETHUM GRAVEOLENS]

This essential oil is good for colic, flatulence, and indigestion.

LAVENDER [LAVANDULA ANGUSTUFOLIA]

Lavender is the most versatile of the essential oils. You can combine it with virtually every other oil in the market; you can use undiluted sparingly without side effects, and it can be used for a multitude of health reasons:

Dermatitis, earache, eczema, psoriasis, sunburn,

muscle aches, asthma, bronchitis, whooping cough, colic, flatulence, nausea, flu, insomnia, headache, nervous tension, and dry scalp. That is just the shortlist.

ROMAN CHAMOMILE [CHAMAEMELUM NOBILE]
Highly recommended for sensitive skin, this essential oil has a long list of benefits as well:

Acne, allergies, dermatitis, earache, eczema, insect bites, rashes, nausea, indigestion, colic, insomnia, and nervous tension to name a few.

YARROW [ACHILLEA MILLEFOLIUM]
This essential oil is not as famous as the two above it, but it does come in handy for helping with acne, the treatment of burns, eczema, rashes, lessening scars, toning the skin, cramps, flatulence, indigestion, colds, breaking fevers, flu, insomnia, and is often added to hair rinses.

2-12 MONTHS
GERANIUM [PELARGONIUM GRAVEOLENS]
This floral oil has been used in the treatment of bruises, burns, congested skin, dermatitis, eczema, oily complexions, tonsillitis, sore throats, and nervous tension. It can cause dermatitis in highly sensitive skin.

TANGERINE/MANDARIN [CITRUS RETICULATA]
This essential oil is labeled as one or the other in most natural health stores and online. This is why I

include the Latin name of the oil. This oil is known to help with congested and oily skin, lightening of scars, a skin toner, intestinal problems, digestive problems, insomnia, nervous tension, and restlessness.

EUCALYPTUS [EUCALYPTUS GLOBULUS]

Well known for being used in vaporizers and other diffusion devices, eucalyptus has been used to open nasal passages and congested chests. It can also help treat insect bites, skin infections, ease muscular aches and pains, sprains, and throat infections. It is also effective in treating bronchitis, sinusitis, colds, flu, and measles.

TEA TREE [MELALEUCA ALTERNIFOLIA]

This essential oil is the perfect substitute for use in killing mold, mildew, and bacteria. It is also used to treat acne, athlete's foot, burns, cold sores, dandruff, insect bites, oily skin, rashes, asthma, bronchitis, coughs, sinusitis, whooping cough, thrush, colds, fever, flu, chickenpox, and measles.

12 MONTHS-5 YEARS
PALMAROSA [CYMNOPOGON MARTINII]

This essential oil has been known to help with acne, dermatitis, minor skin infections, scarring, facials, oily skin, dry skin, intestinal infections.

5 YEARS-12 YEARS
CLARY SAGE [SALVIA SCLAREA]

This is another strong essential oil, but it's good for use in this age range. Since it is a little more potent than the ones before it, I would not recommend making it the mainstay of a blend. Two to three drops should be enough for a tablespoon. This oil is good to help with acne, dandruff, oily skin and hair, muscular aches and pains, intestinal cramps, and flatulence.

NUTMEG [MYRISTICA FRAGRANS]

This aromatic oil is used for helping treat muscular aches and pains, flatulence, indigestion, nausea, and bacterial infections.

Chapter 3

Which Are the Most Powerful Herbs?

GARLIC [ALLIUM SATIVA]
Immune-booster, natural antibiotic, and blood pressure ally.

It's no coincidence that some of the most popular culinary spices are some of nature's healing miracles at the same time. Garlic is esteemed as a medicinal plant all over the world, in myriads of cultures, and is the very proof and poster-child of this phenomena. While it originates from western Russia near the Caucasus Mountains, its powers were so obvious and noticeable that garlic found its way into the cuisine and herbalism traditions of ancient China, Rome, Greece, Egypt, the Middle East, and Europe.

Stimulates the Immune System—Garlic's influence on the immune system is astounding. Not only is garlic's active ingredient, allicin, a confirmed antioxidant of enviable intensity—but studies on AIDS patients have shown incredible immune enhancement after daily doses of garlic cloves!

Such a powerful stroke on the immune system has also made garlic a front-line, long-time remedy against colds, flu, respiratory viruses, and other infections.

Tests and tradition together have seen garlic actively combat infections such as amoebic dysentery, salmonella, E. coli infection, tuberculosis, athlete's foot, women's yeast infections, and even the viral flu.

Garlic's active compound allicin is only formed when garlic is crushed or chopped, and then quickly oxidizes. As such, its immune-boosting and antibiotic effects together can only be attained by eating fresh, chopped garlic quickly.

Blood Pressure and Cholesterol—Allicin and another garlic compound, ajoene, have been rightfully suspected as making garlic a heart-healthy food and healing herb. In daily amounts, garlic consumption helps lower blood pressure and reduce cholesterol, as well as preventing build-up of plaque and blood clots in blood vessels.

Crush cloves for use as a topical antibiotic or anti-fungal on the skin. Crush, chop, or even chew up to even ten garlic cloves a day to experience powerful antioxidant, immune-boosting, and blood-pressure/cholesterol-lowering effects.

COMFREY [SYMPHYTUM OFFICINALE]
Topical magic for bone and muscle aches, sprains, bruises, or breaks.

In ancient Europe, comfrey also touted names like "knitbone" and "bruisewort" for its amazing capability of helping the body bounce back from tissue damage. Applications of the fresh leaf or root, plant juices, salves, or ointments were powerful at mending minor bruises, all the way to speeding healing of broken bones.

Bone, Joint, and Muscle Pain—Traditional herbalists used topical applications on unbroken skin to alleviate pains and aches of the muscles and skeletal system. Comfrey contains rosmarinic acid, a plant component observed to ease inflammation and pain alike.

Comfrey's effects in this realm are the most studied of all—a German collection of studies observes the plant's ability to take the edge off of pain, particularly in those with back pain, arthritis, or discomfort from fractures, sprains, breaks.

Speeds the Healing of Tissues—Another constituent of comfrey, called allantoin, is responsible for shortening healing time in bodily tissues. Using it on unbroken skin over pulled muscles, bruises, fractures, or breaks has been observed cutting down on recuperation.

Comfrey has also been determined as safe for applying to open, minor wounds. A tea or tincture could be excellent for this. Comfrey is also a common ingredient in various over-the-counter wound care creams.

One can grind or chop up the leaves of comfrey and apply it as a poultice to minor cuts or wounds. The same can be done by applying to the skin near fractures, bone breaks, or muscle pain. Comfrey root is also purported to have many healing compounds like rosmarinic acid and allantoin.

You can also use Comfrey in a tea or infusion as a compress for the same purpose. Comfrey oils and salves make wonderful topical applications where there is no broken skin involved.

The crafting of a comfrey tincture or vinegar might help you store it for longer and to apply as a "liniment" in the same way, but any preparation of comfrey should not be taken internally for long periods of time due to the risk of liver damage.

LEMON BALM [MELISSA OFFICINALIS]
Think of a plant like spearmint: lush, plentiful, and cooling. Then combine it with a brush of lemony taste. You have Lemon Balm: an excellent remedy for nerves, stress, anxiety, headaches,

and disturbances that can arise in female health. Its fragrance is heavenly—a crush of the leaves can untangle unrest in just moments. In Europe, this aroma was imparted and extracted to waters, tinctures, and teas to pull away from the distractions of frayed nerves in old times. Its powers were also able to uplift digestive troubles, promote sleep, and support female menstrual cycles. Avoid excess use if you have hypothyroid issues or are pregnant.

Fights Nervousness—Studies have approved the use of Lemon Balm in Europe for low-grade nervous issues. Lemon Balm is very helpful with insomnia, especially if combined with another sleep-promoter, valerian. Some research proved it was just as effective as some pharmaceuticals for sleep problems.

It's been found that topical Lemon Balm essential oil helps calm moods in the elderly with dementia; in Alzheimer's patients, the plant eased agitation and improve focus, making it a powerful nervine ally.

A study of nearly 100 breastfed babies found that Lemon Balm consumed by the mother helped alleviate colic and crying time compared to a placebo.

Even a nice, piping hot tea has been traditionally effective for heightened anxiety and nervousness. Even better, Lemon Balm can help settle digestive upset ("butterflies in the stomach") that arises from the jitters.

Woman's Medicine—European researchers noticed an effect of Lemon Balm on uterine muscle. It is thus thought that it could help allay menstrual cramps, as well as regulate menstrual cycles in a healthier way if taken during certain times of the month.

Hyperthyroidism—Lemon Balm has been observed lowering thyroid function. It is possible that it could help those with hyperthyroid issues alleviate their symptoms.

Viral Infections—European research has also elucidated Lemon Balm as an antiviral, making it a potential ally for fighting colds, flu, and even herpes or supporting HIV.

Teas and infusions of Lemon Balm, taken daily, do exceptionally well—use 1 Tbsp dried herb per cup of water for colds, frayed nerves, women's complaints, cramps, or digestive issues. Essential oils, or just a dab of tea or Lemon Balm tincture, can be added to herpes cold sores to clear them up—or to the skin in other areas simply to create calm.

ASHWAGANDHA [WITHANIA SOMNIFERA]
A nutritive tonic for sexual health, energy, and well-being.

Ashwagandha has been a pride of India's

traditional herbalism and Ayurveda for centuries. Not many may know that this plant with a pungent odor—and roots rich in iron, magnesium, and other minerals—is actually very closely related to our culinary foods of the Nightshade family. These include tomatoes, peppers, potatoes, and eggplants. With such a reputation, some have called the plant "Indian Ginseng" because of its almost "cure-all" capabilities. However, Ashwagandha is more ecologically sustainable to grow and remains a non-threatened plant, while ginseng is neither of those things. This cornerstone of Indian herbalism also has more soothing, affirming qualities as opposed to ginseng's more stimulant nature.

Nutritive Tonic and Adaptogen—Research in Asian countries promotes Ashwagandha as an "adaptogen." Meaning that it contains compounds, antioxidants, vitamins, and minerals that boost the immune system, protect the body from nervous or oxidative damage, withstand stress, and increase the body's ability to create energy and vitality. Over time, Ashwagandha visibly slows "cortisol" levels that lead to stress or depression by helping modulate adrenal output. Thus, this herbal medicine can be a great tonic for stress and depression over time.

Ashwagandha extracts have been shown to influence chronic inflammation beneficially and heal pain from osteo and rheumatoid arthritis.

Due to its high iron levels, especially,

Ashwagandha can be very nourishing, especially for those with anxiety, depleted digestive systems, or anemia.

Sexual Health—Not only has this powerful Asian plant evidenced boosts in energy and well-being, but sexual health also appears to benefit particularly from Ashwagandha. A trial of about 100 adults given the herb or the placebo showed improvement not only in energy levels but libido and sexual energy as well!

Thyroid Health—Evidence highly suggests that Ashwagandha stimulates thyroid activity. It could thus be beneficial for those with hypothyroid problems—but should be contraindicated in those with hyperthyroidism or who take thyroid-increasing medication.

Home Remedy Use—Drink an Ashwagandha infusion or tea up to 3 times per day, using about 1 tsp of the root. Tinctures and supplements are also popularly used with this Asian herb for more convenience in daily regimens.

WHAT FOODS DIDN'T AMERICANS EAT?
ALOCASIA, SABILA, LALOI
- The latex of the inner leaves is poisonous, although it is often used effectively on burns, cuts and to reduce scarring. Most not be ingested.

AMARYLLIS
- Family: amaryllidaceae.

- Amaryllis, naked lady lily, taraco doble, beladonn lily.

- The bulb is poisonous.

- The flower is lovely.

- Requires partial shade and lots of water.

CROTALARIA RETUSA
- Family: leguiosae yellow lupine

- Whole plant has very serious poisons with disastrous effects on horses, chickens, livestock, even humans.

CROTALARIA SPECTABILIS
- Family: leguminosae showy crotalaria.

- Extremely harmful to humans and animals.

- Causes cirrhosis of the liver at the very least.

CROTALARIA VERRUCOSA
- Family leguminosae blue rattleweed.

- Useage causes liver failure and cancer.

CROTON ASTROITES

- Family: euphorbiaceae maran.

- Violent purgative and major skin irritant blisters the skin, and induces skin tumors.

CROTON BETULINUS

- Family: euphorbiaceae broombush.

- Major irritant internally or external.

- This striking-looking plant has several varieties. All are colorful but some of its parts are injurious to the skin, especially if bruised, cut, or scratched.

- Caution should be applied when planting, pruning or cutting clippings.

- It has no fruit to tempt the unwary.

WHAT YOU NEED TO KNOW!

Thomsonianism is a term used in the name of Samuel Thomson, who raised his voice against invasive treatments and advocated in favor of herbal use of medicine, which is more natural and safe. Samuel Thomson was an American. The medical system of the 16th century has its basis in the ideology of Samuel Thomson, and it is, therefore, reasonable to say that the American system of medicine was herbal medicine until modern western medicine came to the world.

Many times during the western medical history, art and science came hand in hand and collaborated to make a belief system which was driven by vital forces.

Physiomedicalist is a terminology used in western medicine for those who believed that some symptoms of illnesses have a positive impact on these vital forces, and some have negative impacts.

All these philosophies with some others which were prevailed and grown in western medicine culture were using herbs as a source of medical cure to the illnesses of human being, and there is no doubt to say that herbalism is the primary driving force in the growth of western medical culture and modern medicine. Natural remedies to treat the disease were more successful in this context, and invasive procedures were thought of as taboo. Mind, body, and spirit were used to be treated as a whole, and there was a significant shift in holistic medicine due to herbalism principles in western medicine.

It was thought that illnesses or diseases are due to an imbalance in natural equilibrium in the body, and this balance has to be maintained to treat the person and achieving maximum health. As discussed in the above context, it is clearly proven that western medicine culture has some fundamental basis, which is quite similar to Chinese traditional medicine and other sources of medicinal growth. So, it is essential to say that nature always played a pivotal role in anchoring the balance of life and death, and this equilibrium of nature is most important to maintain if complete health is required. Herbs are the most natural source of medicine, and the curative capacities of herbs are superior to artificially made substances, which can have more side effects than benefits.

It is also vital that the body's natural capacity to cope up with illnesses is highly essential to maintain this natural equilibrium. Herbalism is believed that by providing some natural resources yielded from the herbs, the body's capability to cope with the stress related to illness can be enhanced to many folds. This is much similar to the self-heal theory of Chinese traditional medicine, which is also used by western traditional medicine experts. From menopause to liver disorders, everything can be cured by herbs. Lignans and phytosterols are essential in providing the cooling and buffering effects on the liver and thus reduce the chances of getting cirrhosis and many other hepatic abnormalities. Isoflavones and phytosterols are essential compounds to boost the endocrinal functions of the human body. Patience is required when practicing herbalism because without patience, there will be no effect on any drug. Herbs are grown with time and in care and compassion. Similarly, it is essential to seek patience when using them for health. Time is always required to boost the inherent capabilities of a body to channel the self-healing impacts. Herbal medicine may take longer than allopathic chemical compounds to heal some illness, but the side effects associated with the right herbs are very less than synthetic and artificial compounds. This makes herbal medicine a treatment of choice in many cases.

Chapter 4

Remedies for Common Ailments

ANXIETY

No one likes to feel stressed out or uptight. Some among us deal with stress and anxiety as a part of our daily routine, or even as symptoms of larger diagnosed nervous disorders that can disrupt well-being. Maybe try some of the following remedies:

Alfalfa—Provides nutrition for those so nervous and stressed out that it interferes with eating habits. Eat leaves or sprouts raw or in a hot infusion over long term.

Ashwagandha—Like Alfalfa is a nutritive tonic for digestion wrecked by anxiety and nerves. Roots and berries in a hot infusion daily, or a fixed syrup, over the long term.

Lemon Balm—Helps calm acute instances of nervousness or anxiety. Helps whether in tea or tincture form, as long as the herb is fresh.

Nettles—Nutritive qualities strengthen those weak from stress or adrenal fatigue. Fresh or dried leaves from non-flowering plant top in a thick infusion every day or cooked as greens over the long term.

ASTHMA

Asthma is a respiratory disorder. People suffering from a bout of asthma find it difficult to breathe properly. Muscular spasm makes it difficult for them to get rid of mucus by coughing.

Much concern is being expressed about asthma today, but, of course, it is by no means a new disease. There were several folk remedies that were given to try and alleviate the symptoms. One old country remedy was for sufferers of asthma to drink a pint of cold water every morning.

They were also advised to take a cold bath every morning.

Not all remedies advised the drinking of water. Another one advised the drinking of apple water, which is described under the apple. Yet another remedy puts its faith in a drink made from licorice. An ounce of stick licorice was cut into slices.

This was soaked in a quart of water and was to be drunk when the asthma sufferer was having a worse bout than usual. Another remedy advocated drinking a pint of new milk every morning and evening.

An infusion made with agrimony was also recommended.

Another drink involved slicing one pound of sliced garlic, macerating it in a dish containing two pints of boiling water, and leaving it for twelve hours. The liquid was then strained, and sugar was added. One teaspoonful of this liquid was to be taken.

Another folk cure involved boiling equal quantities of caraway seeds and fennel seeds in vinegar. Some garlic was then added, and when the liquid had cooled and been strained, honey was added. A teaspoonful of this was to be taken as required.

A teaspoon of chopped thyme was also recommended for the relief of symptoms of asthma. A small amount of lemon juice taken in water before a meal was also thought to be of help, as was cider vinegar. Tea was also held to have curative powers with regard to asthma, and a tea made from rosemary was thought to relieve the bronchial spasm common in asthma.

Carrots taken internally were thought to have expectorant properties. Because of this, people suffering from asthma were advised to eat carrots in order to expel mucus.

Asthma sufferers were also advised to inhale the steam from a combination of boiling water and chamomile.

Food that was easily digestible was recommended. Eating ripe fruits, whether baked, boiled, or roasted, was meant to be good for asthma. An alternative form of food advocated for asthma was thin bread and butter spread with minced garlic. Somewhat less palatable was something else recommended to be eaten as a cure for asthma.

This was a handful of spider webs rolled into a ball.

Other herbs thought to be useful in the treatment of asthma included burdock, butterbur, horseradish, lovage, mullein, valerian, and white horehound.

AWFUL BREATH

Avens, dill, and peppermint were used as a cure for halitosis or bad breath.

Halitosis may be caused by some disorder of the stomach.

To avoid this, one suggested remedy involved

taking a powder containing powdered vegetable charcoal and bicarbonate of soda.

BACK PAIN

An old remedy for backache involved making a poultice from hot aniseed and nettle leaves and applying it to the painful area of the back. Another cure involved massaging with comfrey.

CONSTIPATION

When you haven't "gone" for a day or two, and it's getting uncomfortable, a few herbs might be able to help you get going. Try the following selections out. If you experience constipation for longer than a week, however, check-in with your doctor and don't depend exclusively on herbs.

Plantain—Take several leaves and seeds from this easy-to-find plant, chop them up, and steep them in cold water for a day. If you like—set the sun-tea on the windowsill for a day to help gently extract the plant's mucilage. Drink two times a day until you see improvement. Also: try adding leaves to a smoothie or juice blend.

Aloe Vera—Aloe juice, which is easy to find at grocery stores, is purported to have a mild laxative effect and detoxifying influence on the gut. Try some Aloe juice—but avoid taking Aloe leaf, gel, or other parts internally for constipation. The painful side effects are unpleasant and often not worth the trouble.

COUGHS

These most common maladies can be healed and assisted by the most common of herbs. Next time you or a loved one catch cold, try these out to see if they cut down on the duration of your illness. Science says they could work!

Echinacea—Make several cups of hot infusion from the leaves, flowers, and roots to be taken every 2 hours while sick. Or, opt for a dose of Echinacea tincture or capsule every 2 hours.

Elder—Boil or simmer a Tbsp. of dried, ripe berries in water for colds or flu with fever. A cold-steeped juice is very medicinal as well, packed with Vitamin C. Take tea, tincture, or supplement freely throughout the duration of your illness.

Garlic—Crush, chop, chew (yes, chew), then immediately swallow up to 10 cloves of Garlic per day while you have a cold or flu. Try following each clove with a glass of plant-based milk like almond, rice, or soy. During the length of your cold, you might find that loved ones do not want to come near you. Garlic teas or tinctures won't do you much good!

DEPRESSION

In folk medicine, depression was treated by oats. Other remedies included mustard, cloves, rosemary, cardamom, rose, dock, yarrow, thyme, lavender, and balm.

DIGESTION

There were various natural substances that were thought to aid digestion. These included ginger, cinnamon, peppermint, pepper, mustard, apple, and barley.

Other aids to digestion were garlic, onion, parsley and cardamom, chamomile, dandelion, burdock, nettle, sage, thyme, rosemary, yarrow, and lavender.

Lemon balm, hawthorn, eucalyptus, and myrrh have also been used to aid and stimulate digestion. Lemon, although it is generally regarded as an acid, was thought to be helpful in some digestive problems. The juice of raw potato was also used, as were ginger and cider vinegar.

An old folk remedy involved the use of white mustard.

ANOTHER WAS BASED ON OATS.

Peppermint has been used in connection with digestive disorders for a long time. Olive oil, chamomile, marigold, balm, and meadowsweet were also thought to be effective.

FEVER

Substances that reduce fever are known as febrifuges. In herbal medicine, these included aconite, avens, balm, blackcurrant, bogbean, and boneset.

Also used in feverish illnesses were angelica, betony, borage, catnip, and cowslip. Feverfew, lilac, and meadowsweet were also recommended treatments, as were poppy, sage, white horehound, and yarrow.

Cinnamon, watercress, honey, vinegar, pepper, lemon, and apple were used to help cure feverish illnesses.

Cloves, parsley, plantain, and chamomile also played a part, as did burdock, nettle, rosemary, rose, marigold, yarrow, lavender, balm, hawthorn, meadowsweet, peppermint, and eucalyptus.

Boneset—Before modern medicine, Boneset was relied on to combat Dengue fever and Malaria, two dangerous febrile conditions. Use the dried leaves of this plant in a hot infusion, 2-3 times a day, while sick with cold or flu with fever.

Elder—Elder has been observed supporting the body's own fever conditions, which produce inflammation to kill bacteria or viruses. Make hot infusions of ripe Elderberry tea, and drink freely while experiencing feverish symptoms.

INSOMNIA

Sleep disturbance can be the result of other nervous conditions. You might be wound up tight with anxiety or heavy with thoughts from depression, with sleep always just out of reach. Try these herbs that classically bring you calm, peaceful dreams.

Lemon Balm—Take a tincture or a hot tea of this fresh herb ½ to 1 hour before bed. It might soothe not only depression or anxiety but get you some rest.

Valerian—For really wound-up, mind-racing nights, Valerian does the trick—often with more power than Lemon Balm. However, try the two together to increase your chances: they are a common blend. Tea, tincture, or supplement work great.

Honey in milk with a pinch of nutmeg or cinnamon taken before going to bed was a well-known cure for insomnia.

A teaspoon of honey on its own was also recommended or honey with cider vinegar.

Hops have been used as a cure for insomnia since the Middle Ages. Chamomile was known as a relaxant and was a common cure for sleeplessness, as were lavender and lemon balm. Hawthorn was also thought conducive to sleep, and rosemary was an old folk cure for insomnia.

Poppy and valerian were also used to induce sleep, as were skullcap and woodruff. Dandelion, dill, and peppermint were also used.

Eating onions at bedtime was also a recommended cure.

Either stewed Spanish onions or ordinary raw onions would do, and two or three of them were to be taken. Onion soup or onion jelly was a suggested alternative. Onion jelly was made by shredding onions and cooking them in a little stock until the onions were tender. Boiling water and a squeeze of lemon were added, and the mixture cooked together.

Mattresses were sometimes stuffed with oat husks as a cure for insomnia.

DIARRHEA

Opposite of constipation, diarrhea makes for another unpleasant digestive reality. Luckily, most cases of diarrhea are incredibly easy to support and treat with herbs. If you experience chronic diarrhea for longer than a week, however, check-in with your doctor—especially if herbs aren't helping. It could be dangerous not to.

Goldenseal—If you are worried that your diarrhea is caused by amoebic dysentery, parasites, food poisoning, or digestive infection, Goldenseal will save the day. Keep in mind: this plant will help destroy the diarrhea-causing infection, but not alleviate the diarrhea itself. Take it as a tea, tincture, or supplement.

Plantain—This plant happens to be good for both constipation and diarrhea. Take several leaves and seeds, chop them up, and steep them in cold water for a day—or add them to a smoothie or juice. If you like—set the sun-tea on the windowsill for a day to help gently extract the plant's mucilage. Drink two times a day until you see improvement.

HEADACHES

Ginger—This especially comes in handy for allergy, sinus-headaches with lots of inflammation. Eat a meal with lots of ginger, sip a ginger ale, or enjoy some hot chai tea (which contains Ginger). Or, make yourself some hot ginger root tea.

Eucalyptus—Dab just a bit of essential oil, only one drop each, on the sides of your temples.

Lemon Balm—For nervous, anxiety, or digestive-related headaches, try some hot Lemon Balm tea from the fresh bruised leaves.

INSECT BITES

Mosquitoes, bees, and gnats—oh my! There are sprays and lotions to keep them away. But what about when they have already taken a bite out of your now irritated, stinging skin? Call on these herbs to save the day.

Plantain—In treating bug bites, this is where

Plantain truly shines. Chew up some Plantain leaf or seed, and put it straight on your bite. Or, dab a little salve or oil on. Feel the pain and itch go away within minutes.

Aloe—Aloe can help soothe inflamed skin around bug bites in a pinch. Use its plant gel, a bit of juice, or an Aloe Vera ointment or lotion product.

MENOPAUSAL PROBLEMS

Nettle was used to relieve the symptoms of menopause.

Sage and marigold were also thought to be of benefit in the relief of menopausal symptoms and were considered to be particularly effective in treating hot flushes.

Balm was considered to be of help in relieving the depression that can accompany menopause. Hawthorn was suggested as a remedy for the night sweats that are a common symptom of menopause.

MENSTRUAL PAIN

Got cramps? Stocking up on certain herbs might make you never have to turn to the medicine cabinet again. The following are tried-and-true, studied, and trusted herbs, even for the most intense of menstrual pains.

Black Haw—Compounds in the bark and root of this tree mimic the effects of Aspirin. Seek the dried herb, or supplement form, at grocery stores— make the dried bark and roots into a hot tea, taken 2-3 times daily until pains disappear.

Black Cohosh—A tincture or supplement of potent Black Cohosh can smooth over the pains that come with irregular periods. For the best effect, take a dose twice per day the week before your period. You may enjoy less painful, heavy feminine symptoms.

Lemon Balm—Calming and cramp-relieving together, Lemon Balm can soothe the smooth muscle of the uterus and really help with PMS. Take a hot tea three times per day while you have symptoms, and menstrual pain could hit the road quickly—along with any anxious, unsettled moods you have.

Motherwort—Similar to Lemon Balm, Motherwort can untangle stress or tension related to your period. It can slightly help balance your hormones and takes away some cramping and bloating that gives you discomfort. Works best in supplement or tincture form, taken 2-3 times per day.

Nettles—Think your cramps are more due to bloating or water retention? Try infusions of Nettles or adding the cooked greens to your meals. It's a diuretic—so it will help you rid yourself of excess water weight that leads to menstrual pain.

Turmeric—A pinch of Turmeric powder added to hot water or food can allay your cramping and your mood. Eat Turmeric-plenty meals all day—or sip infusions at least three times a day. Feel the pain go away in time, replaced with warming relief!

VARICOSE VEINS

A poultice of comfrey was used in the treatment of varicose veins. Marigold was also used, either in the form of an infusion or in the form of crushed fresh flowers, as was yarrow. A poultice or compress made with witch hazel was also used for varicose veins to lessen the pain.

INDIGESTION

Dill, fennel, and feverfew were used as remedies for indigestion in folk medicine. Peppermint, speedwell, and thyme were also used.

Ginger and peppermint were both popular cures for indigestion.

The juice of raw potato was also considered to be instrumental in curing indigestion, as was egg white.

Apple and tea were also popular, and another remedy was Epsom salts.

Cloves were considered to be a remedy for indigestion.

Olive oil and cardamom seeds were also used to treat it, and parsley and burdock taken internally were thought to be beneficial. Indigestion was also thought to be relieved by lavender and meadowsweet.

COLIC

An old cure for colic involved administering a drink made from betony boiled in white wine.

Parsley, peppermint, chamomile, cinnamon, sage, thyme, and meadowsweet were all used in the treatment of colic. The juice of raw potato, cabbage, carrot were considered to be remedies, as was glycerine.

Chapter 5

Native American Herbs

Medicinal native plants have been cultivated from the forest and have been introduced for decades to home gardens. The production and usage of such medicinal plants in modern times reflect a safer form of life for the homesteader community, as well as a safe re-supply strategy for the preppers and bug-out enthusiasts. Although these home remedies are never meant to take the place of qualified medical treatment, it's good to know that you're not powerless if you wind up by yourself. Below is a collection of 14 fantastic plants you'll find in the wild. Others can also be picked up at garden centers and attached to your own private garden for medication.

PARSLEY [PETROSELINUM CRISPUM]

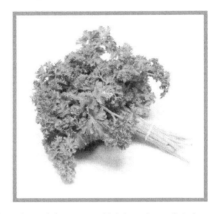

Parsley is a bitter, mild herb, which may boost your food flavor. Some find parsley to be just a curly green food garnish, but it really lets foods like stews produce a more natural taste. Parsley can help indigestion as an added benefit. Parsley is mostly grown annually, but it will stay evergreen all winter long in milder climates. Peregrine plants must mature to be large and bushy. Parsley is an excellent source of Vitamins A and C.

MINT [MENTHA]

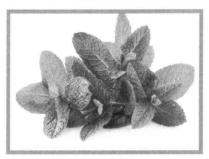

Mint types are numerous. It can be found in cocktails such as mojitos or mint juleps. Perhaps apply some mint to your iced tea for the season. Salt can freshen the air and help relax the stomach. But if you cultivate mint, note it's known as an unwanted herb. Mint spills over the Greenhouse and takes over. This is properly contained in barrels.

DILL [ANETHUM GRAVEOLENS]

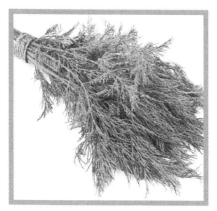

Dill is a great flavoring for fish, lamb, potatoes, and peas. It also assists in appetite, in preventing poor breath, and has the additional benefits of minimizing swelling and cramps. It's easy to grow dill. It will draw helpful insects like wasps and other aggressive insects to your yard, too. It also saves a trip to Santa Barbara Dentist!

THYME [THYMUS VULGARIS]

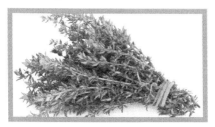

Thyme is a delicate herb in appearance. It is also used for potato, bean, and vegetable flavoring dishes. Thyme is widely found in cuisines like the Oriental, Italian and Provençal countries. Combine it with potatoes, poultry, and lamb. Soups and stews are also flavored with thyme. Thyme is a member of the family of mint. The most popular form is garden thyme with grey-green leaves and a minty, somewhat lemony scent.

FENNEL [FOENICULUM VULGARE]

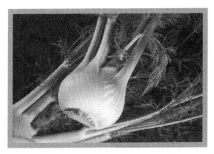

Fennel is highly flavorful and spicy and is a main component of absinthe along with Anise. Fennel is found in the Mediterranean region and grows well in dry areas near to the coast or on the banks of the canal. The fennel's strongly aromatized leaves are similar in shape to dill. The bulb may be grilled or sautéed, or eaten raw. Fennel bulbs are used for garnishing or occasionally added to salads.

FRENCH TARRAGON [FINES HERBES]

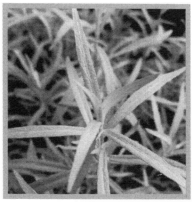

The main component of 'Fines Herbes' is the new tarragon, which is the aristocrat of fresh herbs. A must-have for every Greenhouse with culinary herbs! It will transform an ordinary dish with its spicy anise flavor into a work of art. A little tarragon in a chicken salad creates a huge difference. The sauces, soups, and meat dishes are wonderful. Try on vegetables. Any hearty dish is the alternative.

CATNIP [NEPETA CATARIA]

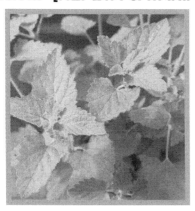

What's more enjoyable than seeing the family cat go somewhat berserk at the catnip smell? Yet catnip is more than merely a stimulant to felines. It may be used both as a relaxant and a diuretic and laxative. When you buy catnip outside, mind your cats love to crawl in and chew on it. Yet having catnips in your backyard can be a disincentive to rodents too.

CHIVES [ALLIUM SCHOENOPRASUM]

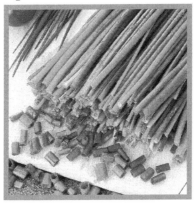

Chives belong to the family of garlic, which can be the best compliment to sour cream. Chives are often used for flavoring and are known to be one of French cuisine's "great herbs." Chives emerged in Asia but were used for about 5,000 years as an ingredient to add to milk. Eggs, fish, potatoes, salads, shellfish, and soups work well with chives. Chives are a healthy source of both beta-carotene and vitamin C.

ST. JOHN'S WORT [HYPERICUM PERFORATUM]

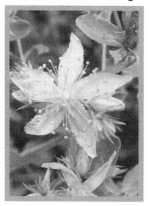

St. John's wort is thought to alleviate depression and anxiety symptoms but should not be considered a cure. It can help relieve muscle discomfort, too. The term "wort" is an Old English word for "rose." The rose was called this as the flowers grow about 24 June, which is John the Baptist's birthday. St. John's wort is also known as the weed, rosin rose, goatweed, chase-devil, or Klamath weed of Tipton. It is a common groundcover in gardens, as it is resistant to drought. This is a well-known herbal remedy for depression but not used in cooking.

BAY LEAVES [LAURUS NOBILIS]

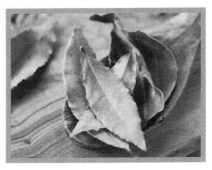

The fragrance of the noble leaves of the bay reminds you of balsam, clove, mint, and some even say, honey! Best known for its use in heart-rending stews and other long-simmering dishes with a very salty, peppery, almost bitter flavor. At the start of the cooking process, add the whole leaves, and remember to remove them before serving. The Sweet Bay is of Mediterranean origin.

WINTER SAVORY [SATUREJA MONTANA]

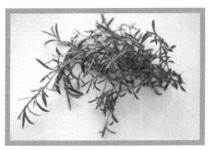

Winter Savory, a deliciously sweet culinary spice, brings an enticing taste to several dishes. Its antibacterial and anti-fungal properties are also used medicinally. Winter Savory, like its summer equivalent, is an aromatic Mint family culinary herb that supplements the strong flavor of seafood, beans, and poultry. During the cooking process, while it loses some of this strength, Winter Savory retains aromatic qualities and is also used to spice liqueurs, creating a beautiful garnish to any salad.

PEPPERMINT [MENTHA PIPERITA]

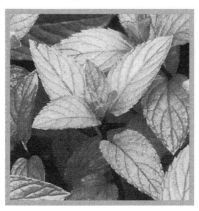

Like other mints, peppermint is popular for digestive help and air freshening. Yet peppermint is also a healthy source of magnesium, potassium, and vitamin B. Peppermint is a combination mint and is a mix between water mint and spearmint. Peppermint oil may be used to spice but is effective as a natural pesticide as well. The symptoms of irritable bowel syndrome have been reported to decrease. Peppermint enjoys ample soil and part shade. It spreads easily like other mints, so try planting it in containers.

STEVIA [STEVIA REBAUDIANA]

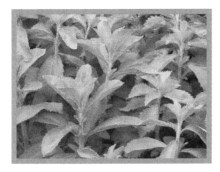

Stevia is an enticing plant in nature and a natural sweetener. The added benefit is that calories don't exist. Stevia is part of the sunflower family, which is native to Western hemisphere subtropical and tropical areas. Though it is a perennial plant, it can only thrive in North America's milder climates. You can add stevia to your summer garden, anyway. Often known as Sweetleaf or sugar leaf, it is grown for its sweet berries. Stevia could be used as a sweetener and as a replacement for sugar.

LEMONGRASS [CYMBOPOGON]

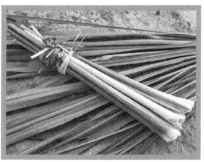

Lemongrass stalks can include antioxidants such as beta-carotene and protection against inflammation of cancer and eyes. Lemongrass has a good citrus flavor. You should brew it in tea, then use it as a spice for herbs. You need to stay in at least Zone 9 to expand the outdoors. Outside it will grow up to six feet high, but if you grow it indoors, it would be significantly smaller.

BERGAMOT [BEE BALM]

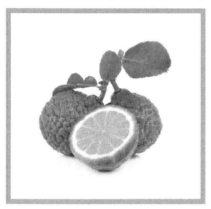

Bee Balm is gaining revived popularity as a culinary plant, making a perfect addition to pizzas, salads, bread, and other recipes that are complemented by the special taste of the plant. Bergamot is minty yet mildly sweet, rendering Oregano a perfect alternative. Bergamot has a long tradition of being used by many Native Americans as a healing herb, including the Blackfeet. To treat small injuries and bruises, the Blackfeet Indians used this hardy herb in poultices. A tea manufactured from the plant has also been used to treat infections of the mouth and throat triggered by gingivitis, as the plant produces large amounts of a naturally occurring antiseptic, thymol, used in many brand name mouthwashes.

OREGANO [ORIGANUM VULGARE]

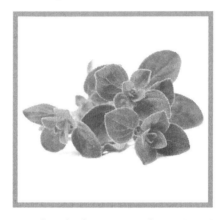

Oregano also belongs to the mint family and is native to Eurasia and the Mediterranean warm climates. Oregano is a seasonal herb which may be cultivated as an annual in colder climates. This is often referred to as wild marjoram and is loosely related to honey marjoram. Oregano is a favorite herb in Italian American food and is used for flavoring. It gained attention in the United States during World War II as troops came home with a taste for the "pizza herb."

COMFREY [SYMPHYTUM]

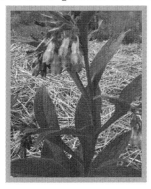

Cooked, mashed comfrey roots used as a topical remedy are good for inflammation, fractures, burns, and sprains. Only don't eat it: a new study suggests that eating in abundance it is toxic to the liver. Root formulations are dangerous for internal usage owing to differences in the pyrrolizidine alkaloid content because they are considered pyrrolizidine-free. While historically used comfrey root tea, the danger of its pyrrolizidine alkaloids is substantial. Therefore, arrangements for comfrey root and young leaf need not be made in-house.

BURDOCK [ARCTIUM]

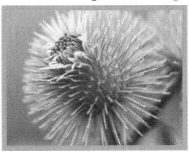

The roots and leaves form an outstanding tonic

for the liver and help purify the body and blood. Most people use burdock root to help them get rid of acne symptoms, and that has a really good impact on a variety of skin issues, such as eczema. Render the dried root tincture in alcohol and drink 10-20 drops of tincture a day. Upon boiling them in water and discarding the water to eliminate bitterness, you may also consume the fresh leaves and roots.

DANDELION [TARAXACUM]

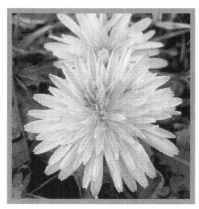

Place one teaspoon of the dried root in one cup of hot water as a general liver/gall bladder tonic and to promote digestion. A root-made tincture can be used three times a day. Some experts suggest tincture dependent on alcohol since the bitter values of alcohol are more soluble. One or two teaspoons of dried leaves may be applied as a moderate diuretic or appetite stimulant to one cup of boiling water and consumed as a decoction, up to three times a day.

WILLOW [SALIX BABYLONICA]

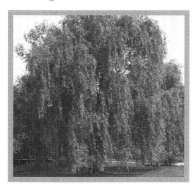

Use one which you can quickly recognize to prepare willow as a medicine. Weeping willow grows in all of North America. Though not local, it thrives in any moist environment, and its droopy twigs and branches can be recognized. Over millennia the leaves and the bark were used as medicine. To produce an astringent, boil a palm with green leaves in one cup with water for 10 minutes. If no other medicinal care is appropriate, soak a clean cloth in this brew and apply it directly to burns, abscesses, carbuncles, and ulcers. Boil the bark scrapings off many twigs and boil them for 10 minutes in one cup of hot water for a gritty anti-diarrhea cocktail. Take a couple of sips every 2 hours, then start until the effects go down.

The bark of many other willow family types, including the black willow, has been in use since 400 B.C. for inflammation and pain management. Black willow bark, a precursor of aspirin, produces salicin. It was once normal for people to chew the pain and fever relief directly on the rasped bark.

ELDERBERRY [SAMBUCAS]

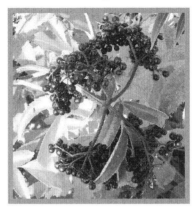

The elderberry is useful when added to the skin while treating wounds. Elderflower is used orally in many nations, including Germany, to combat respiratory illnesses such as colds and flu. Some evidence suggests that chemicals in elderflowers and elderberries may help reduce inflammation of mucous membranes, such as the sinuses, and help alleviate nasal congestion. Elder may have propensities to be anti-inflammatory, antiviral, and anticancer. Dosage is simple. Eat jam or wine made from elderberries only. But be mindful that the raw berries are slightly poisonous. They could have medication reactions with diuretics (water pills), diabetic medications, antibiotics, laxatives, theophylline (Theodor), or immune suppressant medicines.

BLACK WALNUT [JUGLANS NIGRA]

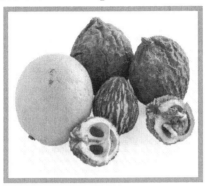

The walnut green husks have many applications in traditional medicine. One teaspoon of the dried green husk content in one cup of hot water can create a terrible degustation, the agent that expels tea. Sip over the course of a day on one cup, and repeat for seven days. New walnut husks on minor cuts and wounds (they also stain the skin like iodine) were used as a replacement for iodine tincture as an antiseptic.

JEWELWEED [IMPATIENS CAPENSIS]

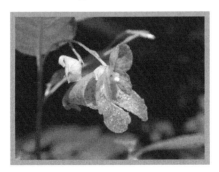

When you come into touch with poison ivy, oak, or sumac, find some jewelweed (Impatiens capensis), smash the moist, purplish plant into a slimy paste, and wash it all over the skin involved. Wash the jewelweed mush away with clean water after 2 minutes of touching. When you can manage so within 30 to 45 minutes of exposure to ivy, you will get minimal or no poison ivy response. While discovering the Jewelweed took more time, you will always feel some relaxation by using it as a shower. Jewelweed's going to cool poison ivy's itch.

MILK THISTLE [SILYBUM MARIANUM]

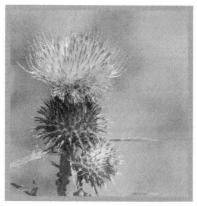

This herb is another great item to pack in your medicine chest. With its ability to reduce inflammation, this herb has been known to have some rather amazing results. Milk thistle serves to boost liver function and, in some instances, has even been seen to reverse the effects of cirrhosis. If you have any inflammation whatsoever, simply apply some Milk Thistle directly to the area afflicted, and you will see results.

RED CLOVER [TRIFOLIUM PRETENSE]

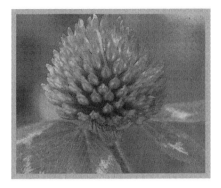

Red Clover is a powerful herbal antibiotic that can greatly boost the immune system. This herb has even been known to increase the red blood cell count in those that use it. Interestingly enough, Red Clover is also a natural anticoagulant and can loosen up blood clots in a rather rapid fashion. This, in turn, provides a general boost in health no matter what you may be facing.

YARROW [ACHILLEA MILLEFOLIUM]

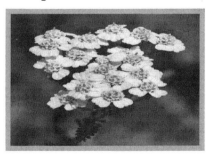

Yarrow is an herb that has been used for centuries; and with good reason. This herb can get to work on inflammation and congestion in the human body almost immediately. This herbal antibiotic also works well against injuries, and as soon as it is applied to an injured site, it gets to work cleansing the injury and promoting the formation of blood platelets for a quick and effective healing.

This herb is a great antibiotic fighter, and its best work is done to reduce inflammation and boost the immune system. Just apply a small amount of this herbal antibiotic to the skin, and you will be able to enhance your body's ability to stand up to and survive all manner of airborne illnesses. Give this herbal Gauche Antibiotic a try!

ANISE [PIMPINELLA ANISUM]

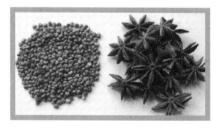

This herb works out just great as an herbal antibiotic, killing most bacteria right on the spot. This herbal antibiotic also works on the urinary system, helping to clear up any incontinence that someone may be facing, and putting the whole body into a kind of detox, almost immediately. One of the best ways to administer this healing herb is to boil it into a nice and tasty tea. So drink up folks, because this Herbal Anise is on me!

CHERVIL [ANTHRISCUS CEREFOLIUM]

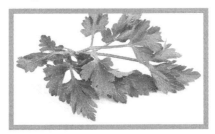

Chervil has a real proven ability when it comes to killing bacteria, getting rid of headaches, and calming upset stomachs. It is the latter from which many a camper has benefited. It is common practice for many survivalists to simply pop a leaf of chervil in their mouth and chew in order to relieve their upset stomach. I have tried this myself and can say that it really does wonders.

CLOVES [SYZYGIUM AROMATICUM]

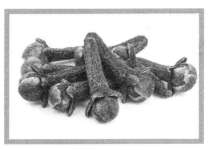

In a similar fashion to chervil, cloves have been placed directly into the mouth of many dental patients in order to kill bacteria and curb inflammatory agents. This herb also works as a mild form of pain reliever and can be used to successfully numb up a bad toothache if needed.

SAGE [SALVIA APIANA]

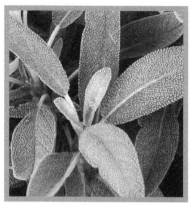

This medicinal herb takes survival medicine to a whole new life in the way that it can successfully reduce all manner of pain and kill bacterial infections on the spot. If you have fallen and sustained an injury, just a very small application of this healing herb will work to alleviate any pain that you may feel. Another great benefit of herbal sage is its ability to treat asthma.

VALERIAN [VALERIANA OFFICINALIS]

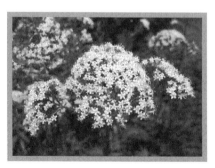

Valerian is also another very popular nighttime home remedies to deal with your anxiety. It contains some elements of mild tranquilizing properties that will almost guarantee you and will get you a good night's sleep. However, without all dreaded and the weird hangover feeling early in the morning that you may sometimes have to get with some other pharmaceuticals.

LEMON BALM [MELISSA OFFICINALIS]

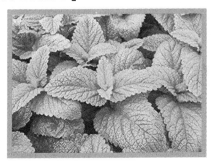

Lemon Balm also is known as 'Melissa officinalis' which is one herbal supplement and tea too. Some studies suggested that the use of lemon balm can decrease insomnia, anxiety, hyperexcitation, and fatigue.

A lemon balm extract should be taken 300mg at breakfast and 300mg at dinner too, which may help reduced insomnia mainly due to a decrease in nervousness and also to decreased agitation, guilt, hyperexcitation, and fatigue too.

CALIFORNIA POPPY [ESCHSCHOLTZIA CALIFORNICA]

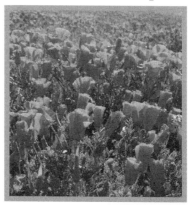

Eschscholtzia californica, which is a tension-relieving, anti-anxiety, sedative, and antispasmodic herb. California poppy also helps with sleeplessness and quells a headache as well as muscular spasm from stress. Some gentle and non-addictive actions are much safer for children and the elderly.

WILD LETTUCE [LACTUCA VIROSA]

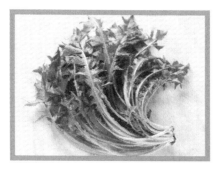

Wild Lettuce is of the species of lactic vireos, which is a mild tranquilizer that may be used for calming a nervous or overactive nervous system.

It is very suitable for anxious children or even adolescents. It majorly helps with insomnia. It is also a general pain reliever and antispasmodic that can primarily be used for short coughs.

ROSEMARY [SALVIA ROSMARINUS]
The herb that makes chicken sing and soups

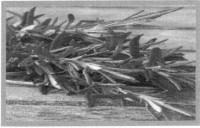

taste wonderful helps treat headaches, nervous tension, a nervous stomach, cleanse the face, and can even help to stimulate hair growth. Great in teas, oils, and soaks.

WHITE WILLOW BARK [SALICIN]

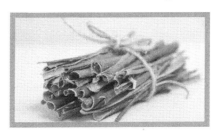

Salicin is an active ingredient in willow barks, and this ingredient is converted into salicylic acid in your body. This bark can reduce the level of prostaglandins that is a hormone-like compound in your body. This compound can increase inflammation, pain, and aches in your body. White willow bark is completely safe for your stomach. This bark can be used to get relief from muscle pains and menstrual cramps, arthritis, muscle pain, and knee pain. It is also good to reduce swelling.

VALERIAN ROOT [VALERIANA OFFICINALIS]

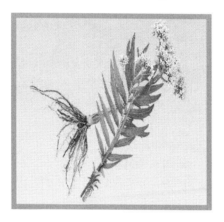

Valerian is an herb, and its roots are used to make medicine for sleep disorders. It is a common herb used with the combination of hops and lemon balms. The valerian root can cause drowsiness and is ideal for those suffering from insomnia. If you are using sleeping pills, then you are advised to treat it with valerian root. The women are suffering from the menstrual cramps and symptoms of menopause; they can use this herb for their treatment. The extracts and oil of the valerian root are used to flavor different food items and beverages.

ARNICA [ARNICA MONTANA]

It is an excellent herbal rub that can be used to cure your pain, acute injuries, and pain after surgery, injury, and extreme sports. This herb is useful for its anti-inflammatory properties.

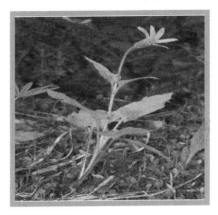

GINSENG [PANAX GINSENG]

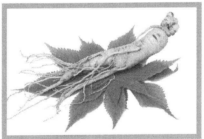

There are various varieties of this herb, and Panax ginseng is the most common variety. It is known as Korean ginseng. Ginsenosides have anticancer and anti-inflammatory properties.

TURMERIC [CURCUMA LONGA]

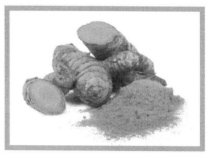

Turmeric contains curcumin that has distinguished antioxidant properties. It has anti-inflammatory, stomach-soothing, and antibacterial benefits. It is good to reduce tenderness by stimulating adrenal glands to amplify the hormone that is useful to reduce inflammation. Turmeric is good for the protection of the liver and helps you to solve digestive problems.

ALOE VERA [ALOE BARBADENSIS MILLER]

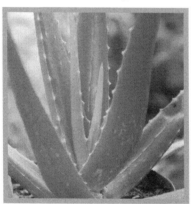

People have been using aloe vera for many

years because the gel of aloe vera is helpful to heal your skin and makes it soft. There are lots of benefits to the use of aloe Vera, such as it is helpful to treat constipation and skin disorders. It can fight with tumors and colorectal cancers. The aloe vera is available in the form of supplements and gel.

The aloe vera is famous for its healing properties, and it is specifically used to treat sunburn and relieve pain. You can apply it to your aching joints to get rid of arthritis pain. The key symptoms of arthritis are inflammation and painful joints; you can take the help of aloe vera to treat rheumatoid arthritis.

CALENDULA [CALENDULA OFFICINALIS]

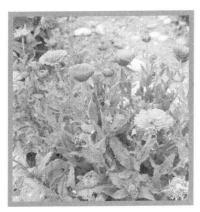

This beautiful flower can be used as a vulnerary agent that is a substance to promote healing. This plant is famous for its anti-microbial and anti-inflammatory properties. It is good for topical use to heat abrasions, treat infections, and infected mucous membranes. It is easy to buy calendula herbal medicines from food stores and apply your wounds. If you want to treat internal infections, you can make a calendula tea with warm water (1 cup) and one tablespoon.

CHAMOMILE [MATRICARIA CHAMOMILLA]

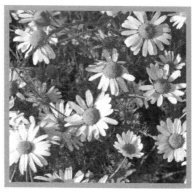

Chamomile was a traditional medicine used thousands of years ago for the treatment of anxiety and upset stomach. The herb is used with a combination of other plants to get lots of health benefits. If you are suffering from heartburn, upset stomach, nausea, and queasiness, then you can use chamomile. It also proves helpful for the sore mouth and cancer. If you have any skin irritation, the chamomile can help you to heal your wounds.

MARSHMALLOW ROOT

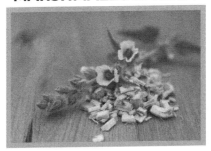

This root is similar to white cylinders and famous for its sweet taste. This herb is found in the candy section of the grocery store. This plant has incredible properties to heal wounds wreaked on your body. This herb is great for extracting bacteria and toxins from your injury. It can heal bruises and burns. You can create poultice with marshmallow and apply on your wounds for speed healing.

PASSIONFLOWER [PASSIFLORA INCARNATE]

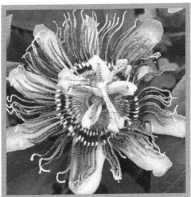

The top part of the passionflower plant is used to make medicine for the sleep problems, anxiety, gastrointestinal ailments, nervousness, and withdrawal symptoms of the narcotic drugs. It is equally beneficial for asthma, hysteria, seizures, nervousness, irregular heartbeat, and high blood pressure. It can also be used to treat skin burns, pains, and swelling.

Its extracts are used in the food and beverages to flavor them. It can be used with the combination of other drugs to prop up tranquility and relaxation. You can combine it with the hops, skullcap, kava, valerian, and German chamomile. The chemicals found in the passionflower can make you calm and promote good sleep by relieving the effects of muscle spasm.

One study has found it has to be as effective as benzodiazepine drugs, but the only difference is without the drowsiness. Passionflower may also help you to feel an emotionally balanced and exceptionally beneficial way.

Nonetheless, if you suffer from exaggerated emotions, then this is by far one of the most efficient home remedies to deal with anxiety, and it needs to be part of your daily regimen.

CAYENNE PEPPER [CAPSICUM ANNUUM]

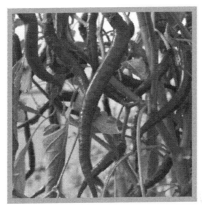

Cayenne pepper is excellent to speed up the blood clotting process at the site of your injury or wound. Antibacterial and anti-fungal properties can disinfect your wounds. With the use of cayenne pepper, the injury may stop bleeding in 10 to 12 seconds. You can mix one teaspoon cayenne pepper in 8 oz. water and give it to the afflicted person.

GREEN TEA [RHEUMATOID ARTHRITIS]

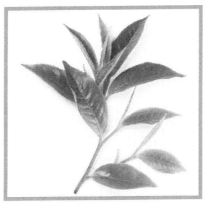

Rheumatoid arthritis can cause severe inflammation to the body organs and joints, and its treatment requires time. If you want to treat it with the help of natural herbs, you can use green tea. Green tea is made from unfermented leaves, and it has lots of medicinal properties. The green tea has lots of useful compounds, including EGCG (epigallocatechin-3-gallate) that can interfere with the particular molecules of the immune system.

There are lots of health benefits of the green tea. By drinking one to two cups of the green tea on a regular basis, you will be able to reduce the risk of break cancer, skin, lungs, and colon and bladder cancer. It plays a significant role in dealing with cardiovascular diseases.

CAT'S CLAW [OXINDOLE ALKALOIDS]

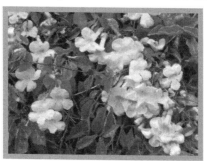

The Cat's Claw is a useful herb to treat stomach problems. It is famous for its exceptional properties to strengthen the immune system of your body. It will enable your body to fight infections and different infections. The oxindole alkaloids can enhance the capacity of the immune system to destroy the pathogens. You can use this herb for the treatment of painful and swollen joints, and the eight weeks are enough to treat different health problems.

ASTRAGALUS HERBS
[POLYSACCHARIDES, SAPONINS]

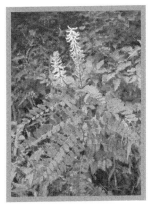

It is a Chinese herb used to stimulate the immune system, digestion, and functions of the adrenal gland. It is a diuretic herb to help your body to fight against different infections. The herb has polysaccharides, saponins, and flavonoids contents. It can reduce the acidity of your stomach, increase the metabolic rate of your body, and encourage the abolition of waste.

The herb can be combined with ginseng to increase the strength and natural defense of the body. The anti-inflammatory properties of the herbs are equally good for fever and other allergic reactions.

LICORICE ROOT [BUPLEURUM FALCIPARUM]

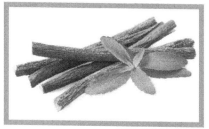

The Licorice is a plant, and its roots are used to make medicine. It is used to flavor foods, beverages, and tobacco. If you are suffering from digestive system problems, then you can use it because it is perfect for treating colic, stomach ulcers, and heartburn. It is also beneficial to use for constant gastritis. It is also useful for the infections of bacteria, including a cough, bronchitis, and sore throat. You can use it for liver disorders, malaria, CFS (chronic fatigue syndrome), food poisoning, and tuberculosis. It can be used with the combination of Panax ginseng and Bupleurum falciparum to enhance its benefits. It is important to produce essential hormones that enable your body to respond to stress.

Chapter 6

Medicinal Plants Used Daily by Native Americans

BUTTERBUR [PETASITES]

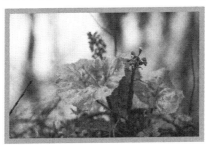

Butterbur, also known as Petasites, is another medicinal herb found in the Pacific North West. It is a perennial plant with thick rhizomes that creep underground. It can also be identified by its leaves that are rhubarb-like. Parts of this plant that are usable for medicinal purposes include the roots, leaves, and stem.

So, why is it ideal for treating headaches? The plant contains certain active substances called petasin and isopetasin. These compounds dampen inflammation, which, in turn, reduces headaches and migraines.

It is found in parts of Europe, Asia, and the USA. It commonly grows in areas that are wet and marshy. You can also get it in forests that are damp and along streams.

GOLDENSEAL [HYDRASTIS CANADENSIS]
Goldenseal is a perennial plant that is low-lying and that has leaves shaped like a palm. A white flower appears amidst every set of leaves, which later on turn into a red berry that gives off ten seeds. The dried roots are used for medicinal purposes.

It is considered a valid option for the treatment of acne because the plant's roots contain alkaloids named canadine, berberine, and hydrastine. These chemicals produce an astringent effect that is very powerful on mucous membranes. This astringent effect brings about a healing and calming effect on your skin.

The plant is native to southeastern Canada and the United States. It commonly grows in hardwood forests. However, if you do not have access to the wild, you can always get them at your nearest herbal drug store.

MULLEIN [VERBASCUM]

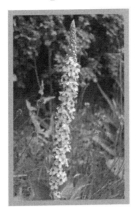

Mullein is a perennial plant that grows to around 3 meters tall. The leaves of this plant are soft, hairy, and arranged in a spiral manner. The flowers are yellow and appear atop the plant, giving it a unique appearance. The parts of this plant that are of medicinal value are leaves and flowers.

So, why is it good for treating nasal congestion? The plant contains tannin that has astringent properties. What this means is that it brings about the contraction of cells and tissues. This helps reduce the inflammation and which in turn reduces the irritation caused by the nasal congestion. This is why it is an effective remedy for nasal congestion.

The plant is found in Europe, Asia, and the Americas. It is often spotted in areas such as fields and ditches. If you are having a hard time finding it, you can easily find it in most natural food stores.

OAT SEED [AVENA SATIVA]

Nervine tonic is another name of oat seed because of its significant impacts on mental health. This is a great plant that is used to treat symptoms of fatigue and stress related to the brain's health. Another benefit of this plant is to use it against many addictions, which are due to the brain's adaptability to this addictive against such as nicotine and cannabis. The withdrawal symptoms of these plants can be so intense that agitated and aggressive moods can prevail. It is a fantastic remedy to treat the symptoms of addiction. Stress is an essential factor that is associated with the brain's stress, and fatigue, and the use of oat seed effectively treats these symptoms. This plant has fantastic benefits of restoring the body's vital energy, which also plays an essential role in preventing stress and mood disturbances.

Avena sativa is the generic name of oat seed, which is used to nourish and improve the human nervous systems. Anxiety, impaired sleep, and decreased sexual performance, which are the secondary impacts of stress, can also be treated directly by using oat seeds regularly. This plant has superior benefits over many other herbs because of having an abundant supply of vitamins and minerals, which are highly crucial for the proper performance of the nervous system.

Adrenal stress can also be treated by using oat seeds in these two types of formulations.

GREEN TEA [CAMELLIA SINENSIS]

Tea is well known and probably the most consumed beverage in the world. The use of this herb for medicinal purposes is well known and has a strong research background. Black tea requires the essential and partial fermentation process of the tea leaves. However, green tea doesn't require these kinds of fermentation and can be produced through the process of steaming the leaves. This process reduces the oxidation capacities of enzymes present in tea leaves, and the preservation of polyphenol is achieved through this process. It is interesting to know that Polyphenols belong to a family of flavonoids which are present 30-40 percent of the total weight in dried green tea leaves. Camellia sinensis is a known name of dried and unfermented green tea leaves. It has a property to reduce bacterial and viral activities in the body. It is also essential in lowering down the increased concentration of lipids in the blood. The potency of green tea to lower down the blood cholesterol level is excellent, and thus it is a beverage of choice to reduce some extra pounds from the body. It is a potent anti-lipidemic agent. Its antioxidant benefits make it a perfect choice to detoxify the liver, kidneys, intestine, stomach, and skin. Its detoxifying and lipid-lowering benefits make it a perfect choice as a natural healer. The scientific base behind green tea is solid, and it is used in traditional as well as modern medicine as a natural source to treat many common illnesses of the human body. It is a super herb in holism, and the benefits of this herb are beyond the capacity of this essential book on holism.

DEVIL'S CLUB [OPLOPANAX HORRIDUS]

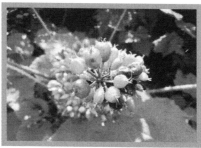

This plant belongs to the ginseng family, and botanically, it is considered in the Araliaceae family. Another name implied to this plant is Devil's stick or Devil's walking cane. Its roots leave as well as stem are used for herbal medicinal purposes in herbalism.

It should not be confused with the devil's claw, which is a plant grown in hot deserts.

This plant is widely produced in the northwest of America. It also contains many attributes of the ginseng family, which is essential to treat diabetes. It helps in curing the insulin resistance. It also helps in lowering the increased cholesterol levels in the blood. The most significant benefit of this herb is its use in weight loss and weight management coach, who knows its herbal impact can help his/her client to reduce some extra pounds in a natural and effective manner. This plant is really a blessing for diabetic patients because it helps in increasing the blood insulin levels and reducing the blood glucose spike after meals, which can be dangerous for pre-diabetics and full-blown diabetic patients. Its anti-inflammatory and antioxidant nature helps in the recovery of cancer patients because it helps in reducing the weight and extra fat in cancer patients, which is caused due to stress. Cancer patients also possess poor insulin tolerance, and thus, it helps in this regard as well.

ALPHA-LIPOIC ACID [S OR R-LIPOIC ACID]

It is also an essential supplement that is widely used in herbalism to cure many disorders and to prevent many diseases. Carrots, yams, and beef, as well as another type of red meat, are rich in alpha-lipoic acid. It has significant impacts on the energy supply of the body called ATP. It also has global effects on the body and can benefit nearly every organ and system of the body, including skin, liver, kidney, heart, and pancreas. It also has many antioxidant benefits, which makes it fit for everyday use. In cells of the body, alpha-lipoic acid contributes to enhancing the power of power grid units called mitochondria. It has been proved in cadaveric studies that alpha-lipoic acid is highly essential in treating age-related changes in the brain. It is a significant health supplement for patients of Parkinson's and Alzheimer's diseases.

It is a very natural type of COX-2 inhibitor, which is used as an anti-inflammatory and pain killer agent in many allopathic drugs. It is also very rich in glutathione and vitamin C. All these characteristics make it a perfect supplement for daily use.

In my practice and experience, my Top 5 Herbs selections tend to cover all my home-healing bases time and time again. Whether it relates to aches, cramps, nerves, or bruises—almost anything, really—I can usually turn to one of my fabulous five without a second thought. All their effects are well-studied, trusted, even versatile and far-reaching, covering a wide variety of ailments, troubles, and injuries. With some luck and practice, I'm sure they'll become your trusted allies, too!

But once in a while, you need another support herb (or two!) to cover your tail. Maybe one of these Top 5 just isn't doing the trick and needs a helping herb to go the extra mile. That, or you've run out your favorite go-to herb in your herbal cabinet, cupboard, or growing at-home apothecary.

What do you do? The answer—turn to one of the 25 following herbs I value as first-rate healers, with just as much study and traditional reputation as my top 5 to support their at-home use! You might not always need them—but knowing they're there, and what they do, will be comfort enough.

ALFALFA [MEDICAGO SATIVA]

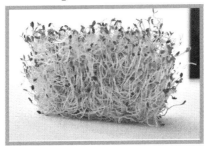

A digestive cleanser, tonic, and nutritious food and medicine.

Enjoy Alfalfa sprouts? Both studies and traditional medicine hold that Alfalfa can have healing effects that combat cancer and digestive ailments. Use Alfalfa by eating it as sprouts or leaves raw in meals, or use fresh leaves in a thick infusion every day. Alfalfa is typically available as an over-the-counter supplement as well.

Alfalfa is a very cleansing digestive detoxifier to the gut. The research observed Alfalfa binding to carcinogens in the colon. European studies suggest regular consumption of Alfalfa helps lower cholesterol.

Alfalfa leaves are a significant source of Vitamin K, Potassium, Iron, Zinc, and Protein, as well as Vitamins A, B1, B6, C, and E.

Never consume Alfalfa seeds, especially in high amounts daily, as they will lead to developing a blood clotting disorder.

ARNICA [ARNICA MONTANA]

A sunny healer for bruises, muscle aches, sprains, and arthritis.

Use the dried flower heads in oils, salves, or tinctures for applying to the skin where muscles, bones, or joints are sore. Or, visit your local natural food or medicine section—Arnica creams and ointments tend to be popular and plenty!

Applying Arnica relieves pain and swelling greatly in bruises, contusions, or muscular injuries where the skin is not open. This is due to observed sesquiterpene lactones thought to activate and intensely fight inflammation.

Teas, tisanes, or liniments (in tincture or vinegar form) can be applied to areas in need of musculoskeletal pain relief. The flower heads can also be heated and bruised as a poultice.

Never take Arnica internally or put the product on open skin, such as wounds or burns. It can cause heart and respiratory problems if absorbed into the bloodstream.

BLACK HAW [VIBURNUM PRUNIFOLIUM]

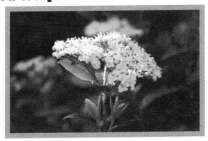

This beautiful bush—with bright red berries and cream-colored flowers—is a cornerstone favorite in United States Southern herbalism. It was once used for all sorts of women's health issues by Native Americans, even for childbirth, miscarriage, and labor. Now, it has settled into the comfortable role of allaying uterine cramps that accompany menstruation—but anyone, man or woman, can enjoy its ability to take away intestinal or stomach cramps as well.

A compound in the roots and stems called scopoletin works to soothe spasms in smooth muscles, whether found in the digestive tract or uterus. It also works on the smooth muscle in the trachea, making Black Haw beneficial for asthma symptoms and attacks.

Black Haw should not be used in women who are pregnant, nor in children under 16 or those with Aspirin allergies.

BLACK COHOSH [ACTAEA RACEMOSA]

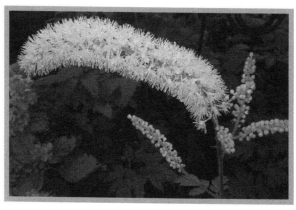

Nature's healing hormonal resource for women.

A native to North America, this stunning plant (once used for snakebites in Native herbalism) has become an important herbal medicine for women today. It contains compounds called "phytoestrogens," which mimic estrogen and fit perfectly in female hormone receptors.

Some herbalists say Black Cohosh is good for women with menstrual problems. It is more precisely relieving for women with low estrogen levels: especially women in menopause. It can provide a natural hormone replacement therapy but check with your physician.

Some menstrual issues are, in fact, due to low estrogen. If you have PCOS (Polycystic Ovarian Syndrome), adult acne issues and/or irregular menses, consider getting your hormone levels checked and trying Black Cohosh.

Avoid Black Cohosh if you are pregnant, and make sure you are taking Black Cohosh, not Blue Cohosh, which can be dangerous. Avoid taking it if you have a liver disease.

BONESET [EUPATORIUM PERFOLIATURN]

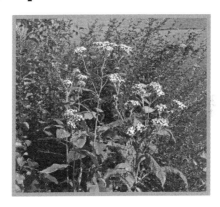

It might be hard not to think this plant has something to do with bones. But actually, its ancient, old-time use was for alleviating colds, flu, and fevers so intense that they literally made your bones hurt! Use the dried leaves of this towering plant in a hot tea or tincture, and take daily for the duration of minor viral illnesses.

Before modern medicine, Boneset was used to fight dengue fever and cases of malaria that wouldn't respond to quinine bark—making it highly reputable to colds with fevers.

Studies claim that Boneset's effects on colds and flu are due to increased stimulation of white blood cells, which help fight off foreign infection.

Do not use the plant fresh, in large amounts, or every day for the long-term. It causes diarrhea, nausea, vomiting, and liver damage. It contains pyrrolizidine alkaloids, much like Comfrey, when used fresh or often.

CINNAMON [CINNAMOMUM ZEYLONICUM]

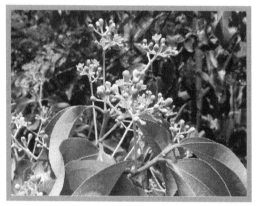

Sweet spice for sweet problems—Diabetes and cholesterol.

Ironically, this spice commonly found with sweet foods happens to be excellent at blood sugar control. Cinnamon is the sweet, powdered inner bark residue from mighty evergreen trees native to India and China. Cinnamon essential oils are available but should not be used internally. Supplements of Cinnamon are available, though it can, of course, be used in meals or in a tea or tincture at home.

Cinnamon affects insulin receptors and helps

create glycogen, a storable sugar. Daily use can perhaps help type 2 diabetics manage their blood sugar levels.

Studies from both Japan and Canada revealed that Cinnamon also helps lower blood pressure and bad cholesterol in turn.

Avoid consuming large amounts of Cinnamon if you have liver issues. Avoid applying Cinnamon essential oil to the skin, as it may cause a burning rash. Do not take medicinal doses while pregnant.

ELDER [SAMBUCUS NIGRA]
Esteemed virus-fighter and fever supporter of the herb world.

If you were to combine Echinacea, Boneset, and ginger together, you would have an entirely natural herbal medicine to combat any cold or flu that comes your way. Add Elder and all your bases are covered! This vivid, dark purple berry is not only delicious—it also stimulates the immune system and combats viruses. Dried Elderberries make a delicious tea or infusion and a tasty tincture. Drink 2-3 cups or take 2-3 droppers a day while sick. Elder supplements are out there, too.

Laboratory studies documented Elder extracts acting exactly like antiviral medicine, particularly for combating the flu. Elder might in fact, help fight any viral or respiratory infection, like colds, flu, or bronchitis.

Elder increases the body's ability to produce inflammatory "cytokines" during fevers, which are responsible for killing infections via the immune system.

Do not eat unripe berries or other parts of Elder plant. All parts, including unripe seeds, are slightly toxic and may produce nausea, vomiting, confusion, dizziness, and fainting. Use cautiously if you have an auto-immune condition.

EUCALYPTUS [EUCALYPTUS GLOBULUS]

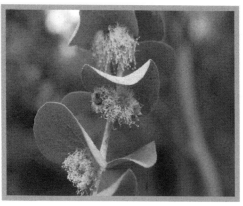

Australia's premier herb for respiratory healing.

A stunning Aussie tree now found all over the world, Eucalyptus has snuck its way into many over-the-counter cough medicines—maybe without us realizing we depend on plant healing already! Oils in the leaves are antibacterial, antiviral, and anti-inflammatory, but the plant is especially best at opening up the lungs and assisting with coughs. Seek out Eucalyptus in essential oils and supplements. Dried leaves are available to make teas, tinctures, salves, and oils for healing as well.

A volatile oil in Eucalyptus, eucalyptol, acts as an "expectorant" and "bronchodilator." These actions help open up air passageways, stimulate productive cough, and produce a thinner mucus that can more easily be expelled.

Eucalyptol is also antibacterial and antiviral, helping kill off illness and infection while also relieving respiratory symptoms. This plant's natural oils are found in many cold-fighting lozenges, syrups, pills, and even chest-rubs.

Do not ingest Eucalyptus essential oils for any reason. Diabetics should avoid use, as it might lower blood sugar. Do not use if you take certain medications. Check with your doctor.

EVENING PRIMROSE [OENOTHERA BIENNIS]

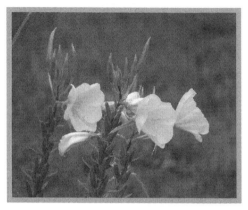

An herbal source for Omega-3 and inflammation soothing.

Because it blooms in the evening, Evening Primrose is given a unique, mysterious name. Its benefits are not so mysterious, though—high amounts of plant mucilage contain Omega-3 fatty acids, making it a target in the herbal world for dealing with inflammatory issues. Evening Primrose is active only in oil form—lookout for oil capsules or topical oils at natural food stores. If you are an advanced herbalist, try making your own sun-infused oil of the seed pods.

Evening Primrose oil (compared to a placebo) helps improve symptoms of inflamed joints in Rheumatoid Arthritis patients due to Omega-3 ability to modulate inflammation.

Like Omega-3 found in anything else, Evening

Primrose helps lower cholesterol, blood pressure, and the risk for heart disease.

If experiencing discomforts, discontinue use. Avoid excessive use internally if pregnant.

GOLDENSEAL [HYDRASTIS CANADENSIS]

Nature's magic, natural antibiotic, and digestive tonic.

Goldenseal's use originated among the Native Americans, who then introduced it to English settlers. Today, it has achieved study and reputation enough to be one of the most wildly popular herbs—though it does hold an endangered status. Traditional and mainstream medicine alike uphold it as an antibiotic and healer of numerous digestive issues. Use the dried root to make a (very bitter) tea, tincture, ointment, or salve. Supplements are available—topical use can help with skin infections, internal for digestive ones.

Goldenseal's active alkaloid, berberine, has proven efficient at combating stomach or intestinal infections like Giardia, E. Coli, amoebic dysentery, or H. pylori, bacteria that cause peptic ulcers.

Topically, berberine helps fight fungal infections and alleviate psoriasis. Its powers also enter the arena of the cold-fighting world—Goldenseal's alkaloid also heightens immunity, which can help fight colds (though it cannot kill viruses).

Do not use if pregnant. Check with your doctor before using Goldenseal if you take prescription medications.

MILK THISTLE [SILYBUM MARIANUM]

A one-of-a-kind liver herb—unparalleled in modern medicine.

Rarely is there a plant out there that can achieve what mainstream medications cannot. Milk Thistle is the exception. A spiny plant, the seeds nonetheless have unmistakable powers on the liver. It might be just the healer for those experiencing liver issues. One can make a tea of the seeds as a home remedy. Milk Thistle supplements are readily available at most stores in capsule form.

Milk Thistle's healing compound, silymarin, prevents toxins and harmful chemicals from literally entering liver cells. It thus protects the liver from damage—even from alcohol, poisons, alkaloids, and NSAID's (like Ibuprofen). Seed preparations are even commonplace in European emergency rooms for mushroom poisoning.

The same compound catalyzes detoxification in the liver as well, making it a candidate for supporting Hepatitis A, B, C, Cirrhosis, and Jaundice.

MINT [MENTHA SPP.]

A cooling, soothing must-have herb for mind and body.

Who could forget Mint? One of the most popular herbs, Spearmint and Peppermint alike are well-used and documented for their calming effects, not just on the nerves and mind—but also on the digestive tract, and for coughs, colds, and flu. Making a tea at home for use every day is perfectly safe, and Mints make excellent, tasty tinctures. Also, seek Mints in cough crops, syrups, capsules, and essential oil form.

Peppermint/Spearmint's active compounds soothe cramps, pain, indigestion, and flatulence in the digestive tract. In the meantime, they also help calm the mind.

Topical applications of essential oils help with nervous pains and aches, even headaches.

The menthol in all mints has found its way into many a cough and cold remedy. It acts as a decongestant, opens airways, soothes coughs, and expels mucus.

Do not apply essential oils to infants or small children. Avoid using Peppermint if you have heartburn, GERD, or a hernia.

MOTHERWORT [LEONURUS CARDIAC]

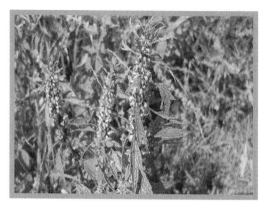

A heart-warming ally for cardiovascular health.

Some may plague Motherwort as a noxious weed, with spiny, irritating burrs that attach to your clothes. Little do they know: a preparation of leaves and flowers could be one of the most astounding natural heart tonics out there! Make and use your own homemade tea or tincture, if you desire. Motherwort supplements are not uncommon either and are an option at natural food grocers.

A Chinese study observed Motherwort relaxing cells in the heart muscle. This then modulated blood pressure, strengthened heartbeat, and even showed the ability to regulate certain heart arrhythmias or palpitations.

The same heart effects have the ability to reduce anxiety, tension, and nervousness.

People taking clotting medications or with clotting disorders should avoid this.

NETTLES [URTICA DIOICA]

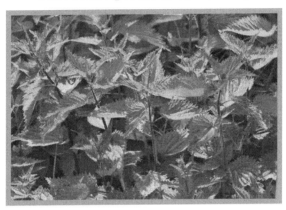

A stinging plant, overlooked superfood, and inflammation healer.

Did you know Stinging Nettles are more nutritious than any plants that might grow in your garden? That includes Kale, Spinach, and Lettuce. Think twice the next time you pull on gloves to remove them like a weed. Keeping those non-flowering, seedless Nettle tops might make for an incredibly nutritious supplement or relief for allergies. Pick with gloves, hang, and dry for 1 hour to remove the sting. Use a tincture or supplement for allergy and urinary issues, or cook up greens from Nettle tops before they flower. Opt for a thick infusion of the leaves for Nettle's nutritional content, excellent for the anemic or undernourished.

Nettles are a significant source of Vitamins A, B6, and C, Antioxidants, Protein, Potassium, Magnesium, Manganese, Iron, and Phosphorus.

Nettles suppress histamine response—great for allergy relief. A noted diuretic, this can be cleansing for urinary health. Studies even demonstrate an ability to reduce prostate growth in men.

Avoid use if you are pregnant. Avoid long-term use as well with diuretic herbs—they deplete potassium stores and lead to electrolyte imbalance.

PLANTAIN [PLANTAGO SPP.]

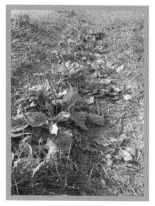

Not a banana—but a beneficial, understated stomach healer.

Plantain is a ubiquitous herb, found practically everywhere in the world. Once upon a time, it was revered as a cleansing, cancer-fighting folk remedy—there's no evidence of that, but today it instead holds the trophy as a digestive tonic, laxative, and topical wound healer. Incorporate Plantain into oils and salves for topical use, or consider a piping hot tea for bowel irregularity.

One Plantain species, "Psyllium," has seeds that are popular, over-the-counter remedies for constipation. They certainly work—all Plantains have laxative action, so give it a try.

The leaves are high in fiber and Omega-3. Raw Plantain leaves added to salads can cleanse the digestive tract and improve inflammation all over the body.

Chew up and poultice Plantain leaves on itchy skin, rashes, bug bites, and stings. It provides immediate relief!

Avoid eating too much Plantain, as it may create an excessive laxative effect.

ROSEMARY [ROSMARINUS OFFICINALIS]

A mind-enhancing, anti-oxidant rich, delicious spice.

Rosemary is probably more well-known for perking up roasted vegetables and Mediterranean dishes. But its history of addition to foods is not only for taste—its antioxidant capabilities were so powerful they prevented foods from oxidizing and going rancid. Those same antioxidant capabilities can be amazing for age-fighting, while other compounds can kill bacteria, improve circulation, and reduce inflammation.

Rosemary's powers to improve circulation are noted for helping stimulate and clarify mental function over time. Coupled with its antioxidants, this makes Rosemary an excellent supplement for the elderly.

The same circulation-enhancing help open up air passageways, assisting with breathing and working as a decongestant for coughs or colds. Rosemary's antimicrobial could also be a further boon for combating infection of illnesses themselves.

Medicinal doses of Rosemary are not recommended during pregnancy. Do not ingest essential oil, and discontinue use if it causes burns on the skin.

REISHI [GANODERMA TSUGAE]

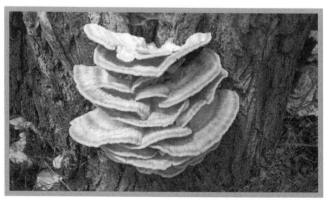

An immune-boosting mushroom for allergies and inflammation.

Most wouldn't think of mushrooms as being medicinal, yet modern research is quickly proving that they are. At the front of this research is Reishi, an enormously gorgeous fungus with species native to both Asia and North America. Adaptogenic, anti-inflammatory, and even anti-tumor effects have been noted. You can use it in a tea, tincture, or extract at home, though most find its taste terribly bitter. Supplements are widely available at natural food stores.

Reishi contains polysaccharides and triterpenes, which modulate the immune system's creation of inflammation. It can thus help with the pain and management of auto-immune disorders—like Rheumatoid Arthritis or Lupus.

These same immune benefits can help with chronic allergies over time, whether sinus, respiratory or even food-related allergies or sensitivities.

Avoid using Reishi if you take blood pressure medication or anticoagulant drugs. Stop use altogether if you develop allergy symptoms.

TEA TREE [MELALEUCA ALTERNIFOLIA]

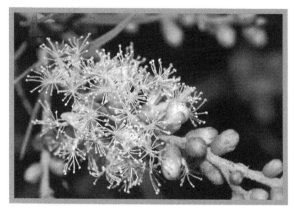

The herbal world's skin healer, cleanser, and protector.

Among herbs, Tea Tree's power as an antimicrobial is almost unrivaled. Originating from Australia (like Eucalyptus), it is now a standard herbal product available everywhere, especially for skin issues and wounds.

When applied to the skin, Tea Tree can rid you of any infection imaginable. Oils in the plant have been observed destroying and inhibiting Staphylococcus bacteria, even antibiotic-resistant strains. Use it as a wound cleanser in a pinch.

Tea Tree makes a wonderful astringent for acne, as it kills acne-causing bacteria. Use a wash after poison ivy, sumac, or oak exposure to prevent the outbreak.

Tea Tree not only destroys bacteria but fungus as well. Use it also for Athlete's Foot, Candida, toenail, and vaginal yeast infections, only topically.

A gargle and rinse (not swallowed) can kill mouth bacteria and prevent gingivitis.

Never take Tea Tree internally; it can be fatal. Discontinue use if you develop rash, redness, contact dermatitis, or allergy.

THYME [THYMUS VULGARIS]

A sprig of flavor for the cough, cold, and respiratory spells.

Much like Eucalyptus and Mint, Thyme too has snuck its way into many an over-the-counter cold and flu remedy. This is probably because this culinary herb also has bronchio-dilating, decongestant, expectorant, and anti-microbial powers. Make a tea of the sprigs, or keep your own tincture for use at home. It's also found as a popular essential oil for topical use and healing supplement for internal use.

Thyme's properties act through thymol, a volatile oil that helps open up the airways and clear mucus. At the same time, it helps inhibit the growth of viruses that causes colds and flu—probably the reason why thymol is also found in commercial cough syrups and lozenges.

Thymol is also the anti-microbial ingredient in some mouthwashes. Consider using Thyme as a mouth rinse for preventing gingivitis and mouth infections.

Do not use Thyme essential oil internally. Consult your doctor if you are taking medicinal doses of Thyme, and you have thyroid issues.

TURMERIC [CURCUMA LONGA]

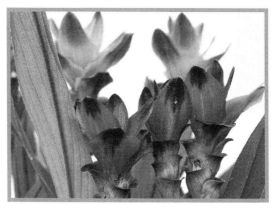

A curry cornerstone that heals digestive inflammation.

Yes, Turmeric is most famous for adding color, body, and deep flavor to curry blends from India. But in the country's culinary and Ayurvedic traditions, the bright yellow powdered root miraculously soothed inflammation like no other. Today, its properties are highly celebrated, respected, and touted all over the world by science and tradition alike.

Turmeric's active ingredient, curcumin, is an anti-inflammatory especially influential on the digestive tract. Research shows that it eases the symptoms of those with Crohn's Disease, IBS (Irritable Bowel Syndrome), and Colitis.

Topical applications have also been seeing helping the inflammatory pain of Rheumatoid and Osteo-arthritis alike.

Avoid taking excessively large amounts. Avoid using Turmeric if you have a blood clotting disorder or take blood clotting medication.

Chapter 7

Most Common DIY Herbal Recipes

Herbal medicine can be made at home in the form of teas, tinctures, washcloths, and oils. Some forms also use external ways of application, for example, baths.

TEAS

Tea is well known and probably the most consumed beverage in the world. The use of this herb for medicinal purposes is well known and has a strong research background. Black tea requires the essential and partial fermentation process of the tea leaves. However, green tea doesn't require these kinds of fermentation and can be produced through the process of steaming the leaves. This process reduces the oxidation capacities of enzymes present in tea leaves, and the preservation of polyphenol is achieved through this process. It is interesting to know that Polyphenols belong to a family of flavonoids which are present 30-40 percent of the total weight in dried green tea leaves.

Dosing of tea depends upon different factors and situations. When used in acute disorders and illnesses, the current complaint guides the dosage. Acute conditions may require multiple doses per day as compared to chronic doses, which require fewer doses for a prolonged time. Herbal medicine incorporates dosage according to the individual needs of a person rather than just treating symptoms with predetermined dosing strategies. It is not essential to stick with a specific pattern of dosing, and it can vary according to personal needs and interests, which is not practice when it comes to western allopathic medicine.

Teas are made from the specific plants of the tea family, and leaves of tea plants are mostly used in this process. However, other parts, such as flowers, can also be used. It can be made from dried or fresh parts of tea making plants, and the servings per day can vary from 2-6 doses depending upon personal needs and tolerance. Sampling mixing the leaves of tea plants in a hot water cup and mixing with honey can provide thousands of health benefits, or it can be made by proper boiling and adding milk, etc. which is called actual fermentation of tea such as black tea.

Tea can be made from hand-picked leaves of tea plant grown in self botanic gardens, or it can be made from pre-designed herbal tea bags for convenience. When aromatic tea sources such as rosemary are used, its steam can also provide a face freshening treatment, which is a common practice in many western and Indian ayurvedic beauty treatments. Artificial or natural sweeteners such as honey can be used for adding more flavor to herbal teas. Stevia teas are naturally lovely in taste. Take a pinch of stevia tea, cool it in open-air, then put it in a freezer bag. Then these bags can be put flat in freezers. When hit, a layer of frozen stevia tea can be break into ice chips, which can be used in other drinks to sweeten them as well as many benefits of stevia tea can be obtained through this process in regular drinks.

DECOCTIONS

Decoctions are widely used sources of herbal medicine in herbalism. When roots or barks of plants contain medicinal benefits, it is hard to obtain extracts from these hard parts of plants, such as willow bark. Decoctions are great ways when the extraction of herbal medicine is required from these hard parts of plants. To obtain this, simmer the herb in hot water pan for at least twelve to thirty minutes on low flame. 1:32 ratio is essential to obtain decoctions from the herbs. A commonly used recipe involves 30 grams of herb and 1000ml of water.

Teas and decoctions are widely used as an herbal source of medicine preparation, and the reason behind using them on a wide-scale is easy to use properties. Just sipping through the cup is all it requires to administer the medicine inside the body. Even rinses and gargles can also be made from these two sources to relieve symptoms related to mouth and throat diseases.

POPSICLES

Popsicles can be made from a variety of sources, and it is an excellent source of reducing inflammation and pain related to the oral mucosa. Another benefit of Popsicle is its incredible taste and ease of use.

ICE CUBES

Ice cubes are a fantastic source of herbal delivery, and they are straightforward to administer. It can be made from teas and decoctions as well. Liquid herbal medicine can be frozen after boiling and rapid cooling, a process called thawing. It also contains pain-relieving benefits, which are very specific with cold therapy. If we add sticks inside ice cubes, they can easily be turned into homemade sweet popsicles. This form of administration is highly famous among children. The ice bags and trays should be labeled accordingly to avoid issues.

BATHS

The largest organ of the body is the skin, which has a very complicated structure and very diverse in properties and colors. Skin is porous and can allow transmission of medicine into deep structures when suitable media is used. Teas and decoctions are also used in bathing to enhance the delivery of medicine, for example, in sauna bathing. Hands and feet can be bathed alone in pots filled with herbal water, or full body can be soaked in a bathtub to achieve the medicinal benefits of herbal medicine. In bedridden patients, a damp cloth with medicinal fluid in it is a smart way of medicinal bed bathing.

Hot baths are essential because they can make skin porous, and thus more drugs can be administered inside the body. Care should be taken when using a hot water bath to avoid burns and bruising. Bathing can be achieved by directly introducing dried herbs in bathtubs or pots to unlock maximum healing benefits. These herbs can be inserted directly in the bathtub, or these can be introduced in porous clothes like socks, pantyhose, and other delicate clothes to avoid a mess. Even loofa made from herbs can be used to be rubbed on the skin directly to maximize the absorption of the medicine through the skin. It is the smartest way of administration, but it can turn bathtubs a little messy and hard to clean.

BREAST MILK

Infants can also use herbal medicine, but the route of administration, as well as dosing, can be very troublesome to decide. A full cup of tea and an ice cube of decoction is a terrible idea when used for infants. We have to decide the safest routes of administration because of the delicate body of infants. Breast milk is a natural source to nourish babies from the nutrients in the mother's blood. Breast milk is the safest of all the routes of nourishment because many complex nutrients that cannot be introduced in an infant's body otherwise can easily be inserted through breast milk.

A mother and her child both can be benefited in that way. Some herbal medicines are really infant friendly while others can be harsher on the delicate infant body, so careful consideration before administration is essential to avoid any kind of side effects. Another significant benefit is to insert potent herbal antibacterial medicine inside an infant to make more him/her more immune to side effects of getting sick from antibacterials is to introduce them from the mother's breast milk. It will boost the natural immunization responses in both mother and her infant.

WASHCLOTHS

Washcloths are indeed a great source to get bathed on the bed. They can be used on a critically ill patient who cannot survive an active bath. In this comfortable way, medicine can easily be applied to the skin, and thus it can be transferred to a deeper area of the body through diffusion. Washcloths can be warm by using hot infusions of medicine when specific impacts of heating are needed, or they can be cold when benefits of cold are needed. It all depends upon personal choice as well as symptoms of illnesses. For acute injuries, for example, brushing and combat sports fights, cold washcloths with specific benefits of ice and anti-inflammatory medicine can be a smart choice to limit swelling and bruising as well as impeding bleeding from fresh wounds. Cold also has anesthetic properties, which make it a natural pain killer.

When used warm, washcloths can stimulate blood flow due to vasodilatory effects as well as a soothing response of the body can also be obtained.

COMPRESSES

Compresses are warm medicinal pastes which are formed from many potent herbs. It is a very traditional technique, which is also caller "Marham" in Arabic, and it is the most used technique in Indian ayurvedic as well. Warm herbs in the form of compresses can stay longer than washcloths on the skin and can be a great source of constant delivery of herbal medicine. The feeling of warmth is soothing itself, and it also helps in reducing muscle spasm when applied. It also helps in vasodilation in specific areas to speed up recovery. Some herbs are delightful in fragrance and thus can provide the body with an unusual odor. Any natural fiber, a cloth with pores or muslin bag, can be used to form compresses from medicinal herbs. In traditional herbal medicine, compresses were formed by putting them in direct sunlight to get the effects of warmth. In modern days, ovens can be used to achieve the temperature and thus applied to the skin in comfortable ways. Microwaving should be avoided when other natural sources are available because of the health hazards of artificial heating. Different and multiple layers are also used over single compress to achieve maximum absorption as well as the mixing of herbs. It also protects from overheating and bruising.

POULTICES:

Poultice or Marham is a type of herbal medicine that is applied to skin sores and wounds directly to achieve healing at maximum pace and to unlock bactericidal and anti-inflammatory benefits. It is an excellent source of delivering medicine from the skin to other, more profound layers of the body. Again, it is popular form of medicine in traditional Chinese, Indian, and Muslim herbalism. It is so easy to apply the poultices that it can be applied to gums in the mouth as well as on lips to treat symptoms of herpes and other STDs. Any type of fresh, damp, or dried herbs can be used to make poultices. Another effective way to apply them is to keep them on wounds for more extended periods to achieve maximum absorption. It is a widely used method of administration in herbal dentistry because it is by far the safest method to be used in the oral cavity. A poultice can be left overnight or longer in the mouth to avoid bruising and sores in the mouth. It will also help in improving the freshness of mouth and thus promoting the better odor in breath. It is essential to know the dosage of the herb in a poultice. A poultice is a damp or less wet type of medication, more like a paste which can be made by just mixing water, tea, or decoction in a dried paste of herb. A mixture of different herbs can also be used to make a poultice to unlock many benefits hidden in these different herbs. It is a fantastic strategy that is used by many herbalists. For example, an analgesic herb containing pain killer properties can be mixed with antioxidant, anti-inflammatory, or any type of bactericidal herb to achieve all these impacts by a single use of poultice. A great recipe involves the use of herbal tea with blueberry along with willow to unlock the actions of all these three herbs in a single poultice.

TINCTURES

Tinctures are drops of herbs in liquid form, which are combined in 80-95% of the alcohol base. The most crucial benefit of this type of administration is the very long preservation period of medicine achieved by adding alcohol into it. It is such a diluted form of medicine that hardly any side effect can occur. This is the sole reason that homeopaths used these types of tinctures for centuries to administer drugs in human bodies. The tincture can be prepared by mixing herb into wine, vodka, or rum.

A more diluted media such as apple cider vinegar or glycerine can also be used to achieve these benefits. Alcohol-free media can also be used to make tinctures of very diluted quality for those who don't like alcohol to get ingested. Tinctures can be prepared in homes as well as they can also be available in markets. However, the best practice is to make it at home because it doesn't require any special treatment to prepare all these effective tinctures at home. Lay herbalists are famous for making their own tinctures.

Raw alcohol is best to make tinctures rather than flavored vodka or rum so that the maximum benefits of herbs can be preserved. Flavoring is also rich in dirty surfers, which are not the right choice for medicinal purposes. Grain alcohol is the most popular type of alcohol used by herbalists to achieve the preparation of the highest quality tinctures. Vodka and grain are very different because they are made from very different sources. Twenty percent net alcohol should be used when the dried herb is made, and 40% of alcohol can be mixed with the fresh herb to ensure proper mixture and administration without side effects.

Willow bark is known to have high tannin concentration, and thus adding a few amounts of glycerin can be a smart idea for extracting maximum concentration of herb. A tincture is nothing when inferior ingredients are used. Alcohol is just a base in it; however, the medicinal benefits of a tincture can only be achieved from using proper herbs only. A perfect ratio is 1:5 that is 1 part alcohol with five parts of herbs to ensure more concentration of herb in a tincture. This guide is a critical ad accepted in herbalist society all over the world.

In the case of yarrow, we make an alcohol-based. Yarrow or other types of tannin-containing herbs can be mixed with glycerine and alcohol to extract the medicinal benefits from them properly. The next stage is to put the solution in a dark room while keeping the solution in a tight jar for more than three weeks. A proper shaking of the jar every week can also promote proper extraction of the herbal medicinal benefits.

The use of tea and decoction, along with water, can also be applied while making an alcohol free tincture. The final step of tincturing is to stain the solution. The solution is called menstruum, which, while stained, is called a tincture. It is essential to label the jar with the proper name for identification purposes.

These are common and most effective techniques to prepare proper herbal medications at home with much effort and preparation.

INFUSION

An infusion is prepared by mixing the herbs with water or oil and waiting for the chemical compounds to mix with the solvent. This process is known as steeping. Infusion is used when the active ingredients of the plant materials used dissolve used when put in the solvent. Many of the materials used are leaves, flowers, berries, and seeds either in whole or when they are dried and pounded or ground. The liquid is boiled and the herbs are added and allowed to steep for some time, usually 15-30 minutes. The herbs can be removed, or the liquid is strained and drunk either immediately or later.

Conclusion

The fact that you are putting all this effort shows a real dedication and commitment to taking matters of your health seriously. There are many prescription drugs out there. However, it doesn't mean that they are the only options available.

For simple ailments, you can always resort to herbal remedies like the ones we have discussed in this book. There is no need to create dependency on prescription drugs. Going herbal is much safer and healthier most of the time. If you are in doubt, always consult your physician first.

Starting out learning herbalism and plant-based home remedies can be difficult, but I hope—and I'm sure—that this book has been an excellent primer for you to continue your journey, get acquainted with the plants, select which ones work best for you—and to empower healing at home.

There is a lot of information on herbs out there. I have done my very best, with all honesty, in my research and personal quest for the most tried-and-true herbal remedies. If you are inspired, don't hesitate to find yet more truth and information out there on the subject. The world of herbalism is vast and deep—and the deeper you go, the more safe healing, magic, and miracles you'll find!

Thank you!

Manufactured by Amazon.ca
Bolton, ON